NONNATUS
HOUSE

THE LIFE AND TIMES OF
CALL THE MIDWIFE

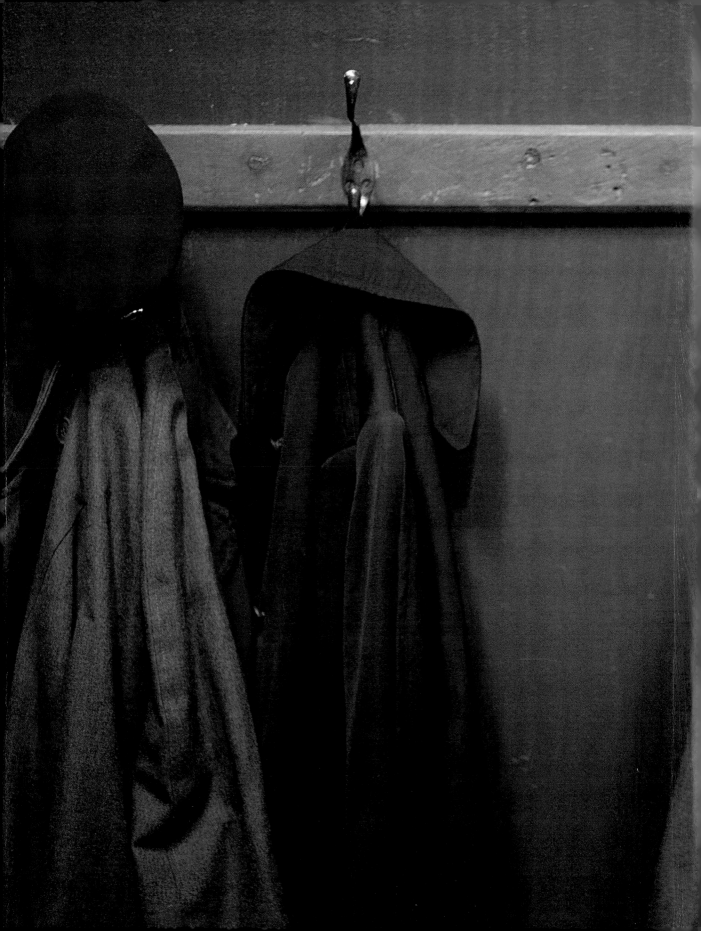

THE LIFE AND TIMES OF
CALL THE MIDWIFE

The Official Companion to Seasons One and Two

HEIDI THOMAS

Foreword by JENNY AGUTTER, OBE

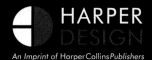

HARPER
DESIGN

An Imprint of HarperCollinsPublishers

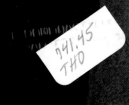

CONTENTS

FOREWORD by *Jenny Agutter OBE*   06
INTRODUCTION by *Heidi Thomas*   08

CHAPTER 1
BIRTH
14

PROFILES
+
THE NURSES
42

CHAPTER 2
FASHION
58

CHAPTER 3
Beauty
80

Call the Midwife Diaries part 1
96

CHAPTER 4
FAITH
108

PROFILES
✝
THE NUNS
126

CHAPTER 5 HEALTH
142

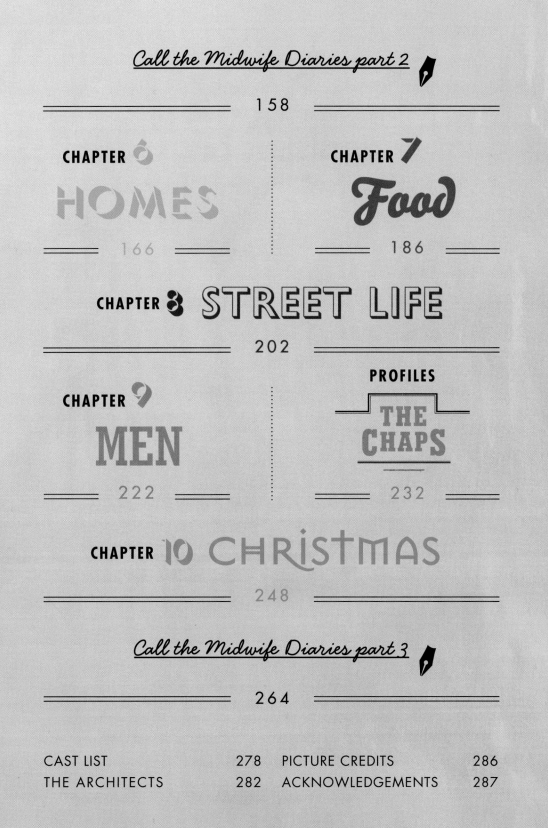

Call the Midwife Diaries part 2

158

CHAPTER 6

HOMES

166

CHAPTER 7

Food

186

CHAPTER 8 STREET LIFE

202

CHAPTER 9

MEN

222

PROFILES

THE CHAPS

232

CHAPTER 10 CHRISTMAS

248

Call the Midwife Diaries part 3

264

CAST LIST   278   PICTURE CREDITS   286
THE ARCHITECTS   282   ACKNOWLEDGEMENTS   287

FOREWORD

JENNY AGUTTER OBE

I was born in Somerset in the 1950s. My father told me recently that he was present at my birth, but as men were not allowed into the delivery room at the time it was more likely that I had arrived, been cleaned up, and presented to him as a neat mewling bundle. Although my parents did not share the same faith, they gave me a religious upbringing. Decades later my son was born on Christmas Day, which meant I had shifts of midwives attend his birth. I thought I knew about the period, religion and midwives and would be well prepared to play Sister Julienne in *Call the Midwife*, but I had a lot to learn.

Time was set aside before filming the first series to learn how to appear adept at being midwives, particularly at handling newborn babies. Serendipitously, I met the real-life Julienne's niece, who gave me valuable insight into her aunt's personality and lent me some

of her drawings and letters. She was a talented amateur watercolourist who always found time to send painted cards and notes to family and friends, never forgetting an anniversary or birthday. I discovered a deceptively strong-willed woman with a great sense of humour who enjoyed people with all their faults, always finding the best in them.

The more I discover about the nuns who worked in the East End, the more my respect grows for these women whose faith gives them an unquestioning sense of purpose. They served their community, particularly the women, at the most vulnerable and intimate time in their lives. Childbirth is always a miracle and midwives are indeed unsung heroes.

My parents went out of their way to make sure that my brother and I were not burdened with any of the concerns and fears they had grown up

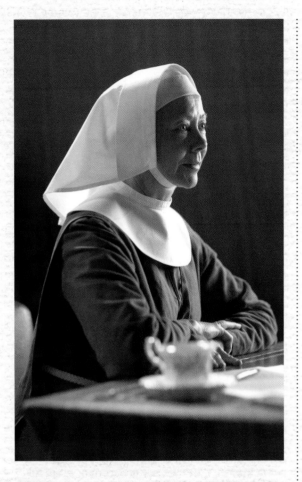

Because many of the characters in *Call the Midwife* are based on real people who lived and worked in the East End, all the cast feel a keen responsibility to serve them well. They are vividly depicted by Jennifer Worth in her bestselling memoirs, and brilliantly shaped for the series by Heidi Thomas, and have been a pleasure to get to know and play. You always hope that an audience will enjoy work that you feel proud of. I was delighted and amazed by the diverse audience we reached and find myself being stopped by people of all ages and backgrounds who want to let me know how the series has affected them.

Costumes and set design play a vital part in creating the mood and helping the actor believe in what they are doing. The creative team working behind the scenes on *Call the Midwife* have captured the period meticulously, paying attention to every detail. As well as sourcing and recreating the furnishings of the time, the production team found small personal items from the fifties with which to adorn tables, cupboards and fireplaces: books filled with savings stamps, old postcards, magazines to inspire the homemaker with advertisements featuring women, neat and feminine with their narrow waists and big skirts, seemingly unaware of the changes that were beginning to give women an equal place in society. Each chapter of this book reveals just how this flawless attention to detail was brought to life.

Working on the series has given me an insight into the extraordinary decade that followed the war, shown me what faith is capable of, and given me the chance to better understand the delicate and under-praised work of the midwife. It has been an exciting adventure, one I am honoured to be able to share.

with. We owe so much to the indomitable spirit of those who lived through the turmoil of war, and worked hard to rebuild our world. The squalid and poverty-stricken area of Poplar and London's docklands was heavily bombed and there was no money to repair the excessive damage or to re-house the many families who had lost their homes. Subsequently, the tenements that should have been torn down and rebuilt remained occupied and overcrowded.

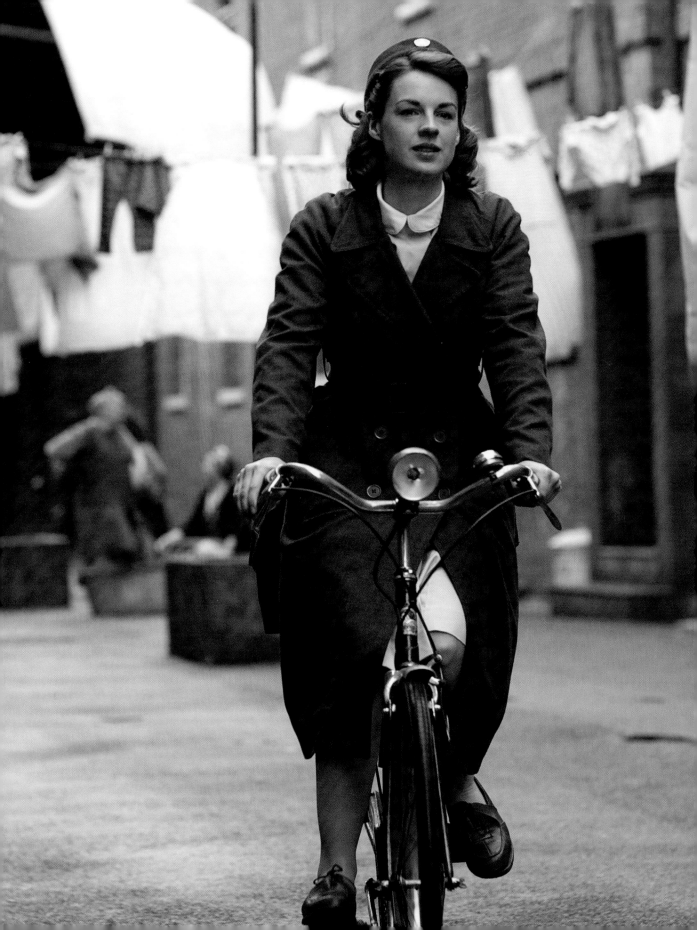

INTRODUCTION

First encounters always linger in the mind. The older I get, the more I appreciate the way the mind seems to take a mental snapshot of the moment. I can still envisage the first time I walked through the doors of my grammar school, the first time I saw my husband, the first time I clapped eyes on my baby's face.

I was initially approached about the book by Pippa Harris of Neal Street Productions, who believed the memoirs of the then unknown Jennifer Worth might have potential as a television series. I was not – I am ashamed to say – especially intrigued. Fresh from the joyful experience of writing the BBC classic serial *Cranford*, I was passionate about finding new books to adapt, but didn't think this would fit the bill in any way. It was not set in my favourite century (the 19th) and, even more importantly, its author was alive and well and living in Hemel Hempstead.

Adapting another writer's work for the screen is a fraught and delicate business – changes are inevitable, and I have a keen conscience. I shudder at the thought of causing distress or offence to the person whose imagination, hard work and talent have brought a book about. While I was writing the scripts for *Cranford*, sometimes the only thing that kept me going was the thought that Mrs Gaskell had been dead for many decades. Meanwhile, Jennifer was not only still with us, but had based *Call the Midwife* on her own, deeply personal experience of working in the East End in the 1950s. I imagined that even the smallest details would be important to her, and that any alterations might prove painful.

'No,' I said to Pippa, 'I don't think it's for me.' Pippa didn't listen. She and I have known each other for many years, having worked on our very first television job together – the series *Soldier,*

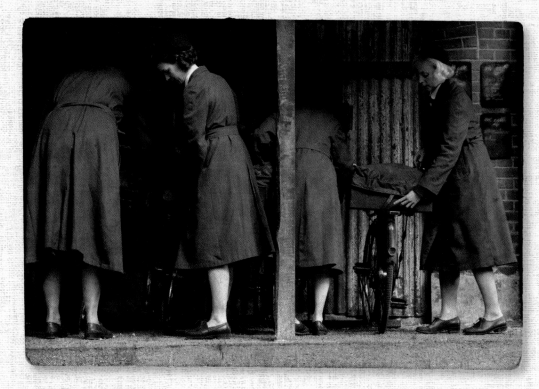

Soldier – in the 1990s and there was a touch of stuff-and-nonsense in her tone.

'Just read it,' she said. 'I know you, and I know you won't be able to put it down.'

'But it's set in the 1950s!' I replied, rather weakly. 'It's not historical, and it's not modern either. It just won't be my cup of tea – I want to do another Gaskell, or a Dickens.'

Pippa sent it to me anyway. I read it, and she was right – I couldn't put it down until I'd finished. I can still recall the weight of it in my hands (this was the early, hardback edition) and the way my wrists ached as I compulsively turned page after page. It was my first encounter with the magic of *Call the Midwife*, and I will remember it all my days: the first sighting of the youthful Jenny Lee, picking her wasp-waisted way through the bomb sites of Poplar; the first batty utterance from Sister Monica Joan; the first time Chummy tumbled from her bike.

Over and over again, I was surprised and delighted by the characters, the stories and the sheer muscular vigour of Jennifer's writing. I have never been sure whether I devoured the book, or the book devoured me, but by the time I closed it and crawled into bed, the die was cast: I was on board, and wouldn't rest until I had brought *Call the Midwife* to the screen.

Looking back, I actually made that decision when reading page thirteen. I know this because my original copy of the book still sits on my desk, and I can see that on page thirteen I underlined a single sentence in pencil, and wrote one word in the margin alongside it. That word is 'YES', and it marked the first time *Call the Midwife* made me cry. In the middle of a crisp, factual description of childbirth in a working-class London home in the 1950s, Jennifer had dropped one beautiful comment that transcended all barriers of geography, class and time. It was this:

'How much more can she bear, how much can any woman bear?'

Those words went straight to my heart. Here, at last, was a book that told the unflinching truth about an experience that defines the lives of women the world over, and has done so for countless generations. Furthermore, birth is something that happens to us all. We must all be born, just as we all must die. It is the one common miracle, an experience that unleashes every emotion we possess. As a midwife, Jennifer understood this more than most, and by setting down her memoirs, she shone an unprecedented light on her own profession.

In turning the books into a television series, it became my privilege to continue the work that Jennifer started. Much laughter was had – and many more tears shed – as the show evolved.

Getting a TV drama to the screen is always something of a journey. As the writer, I travelled alone at the outset. But *Call the Midwife* rattled onwards, a bit like a train, stopping to pick up people along the way. Producers, designers and directors came aboard. As filming approached, we were joined by actors, technicians and composers. There were babies in the mix, and medics to advise us. The challenges were legion, but we were a happy band, and this book is our attempt to share the graft, grind and sheer exhilarating joy of going back to the 1950s to make the show we loved so much.

As I write these lines, the cameras are about to start turning on the second series of *Call the Midwife*. Jennifer Worth died two weeks before we had begun to film the first. She would call me sentimental for this, but I find it impossible not to picture her standing alone on a railway platform, having got off the train several stations too soon.

Ours was an unusual friendship. Jennifer was bossy and I am stubborn, so it could have been a disaster. When we were first introduced, each of us was quite rightly nervous of the other. But in that rare way that happens when minds truly meet, we soon bypassed all the niceties

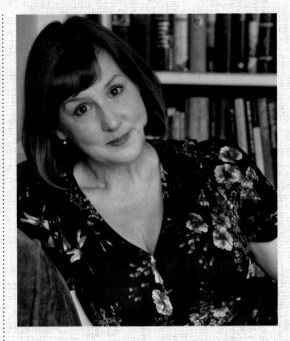

and joined forces. That was that; we were in it together. And we still are.

On my desk, tucked into my very first copy of *Call the Midwife*, is the final letter Jennifer wrote to me. It contains some thoughts on the last script she was well enough to read. She ends, in her elegant spidery hand, with the words, 'I leave it to you with confidence.'

But *Call the Midwife* is not mine, and I do believe that deep down Jennifer never really felt that it was wholly hers either. She always insisted that, in the books, she was simply bearing witness to the lives of others. In writing the television series, I followed her example and tried to do the same. Because birth is in the possession of humanity itself, and from our very first breath, these are stories we all share.

Heidi Thomas

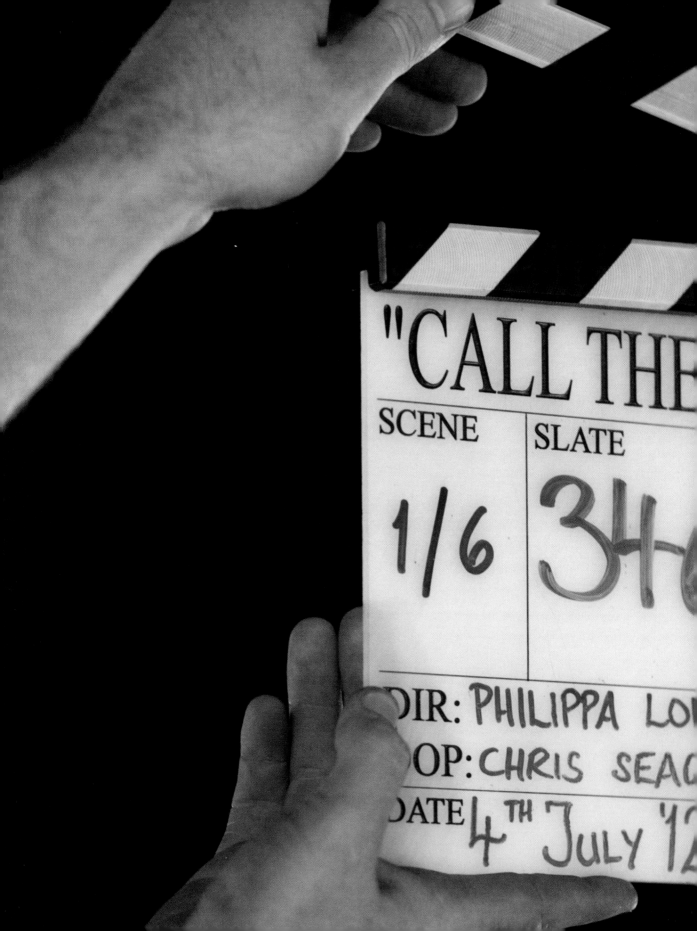

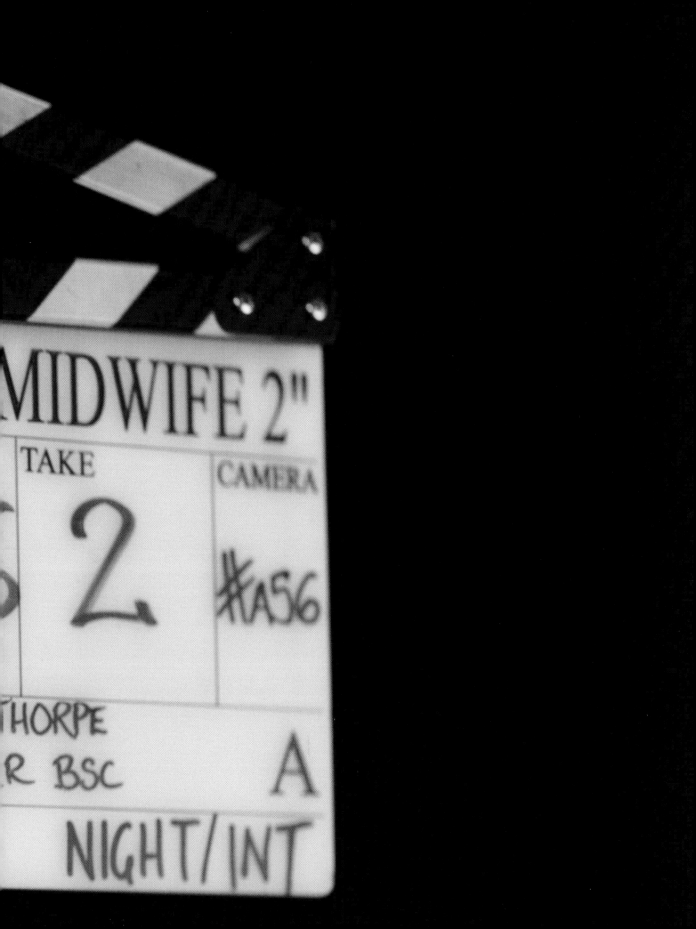

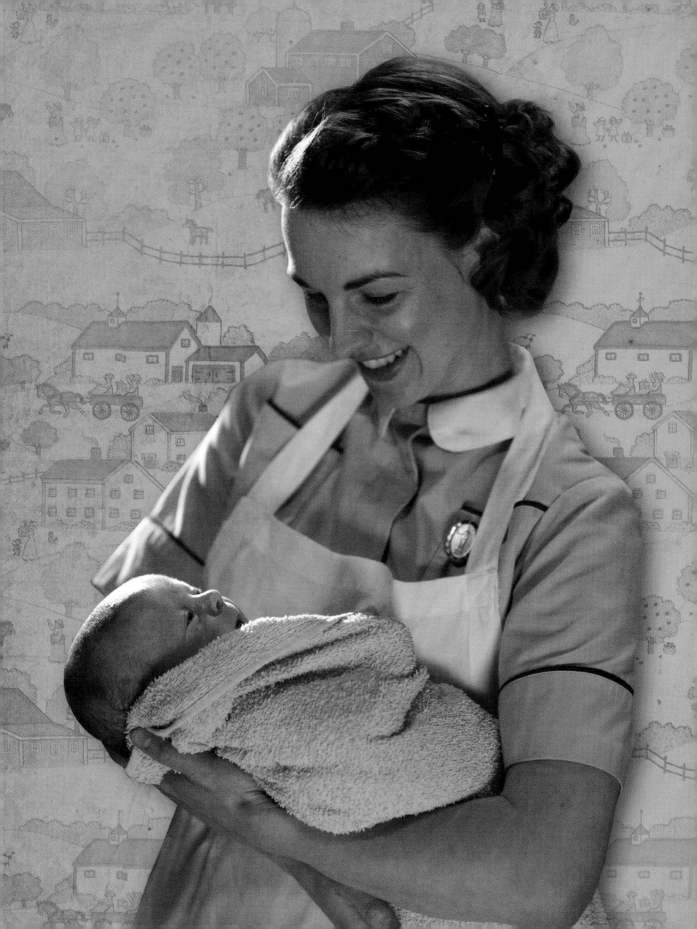

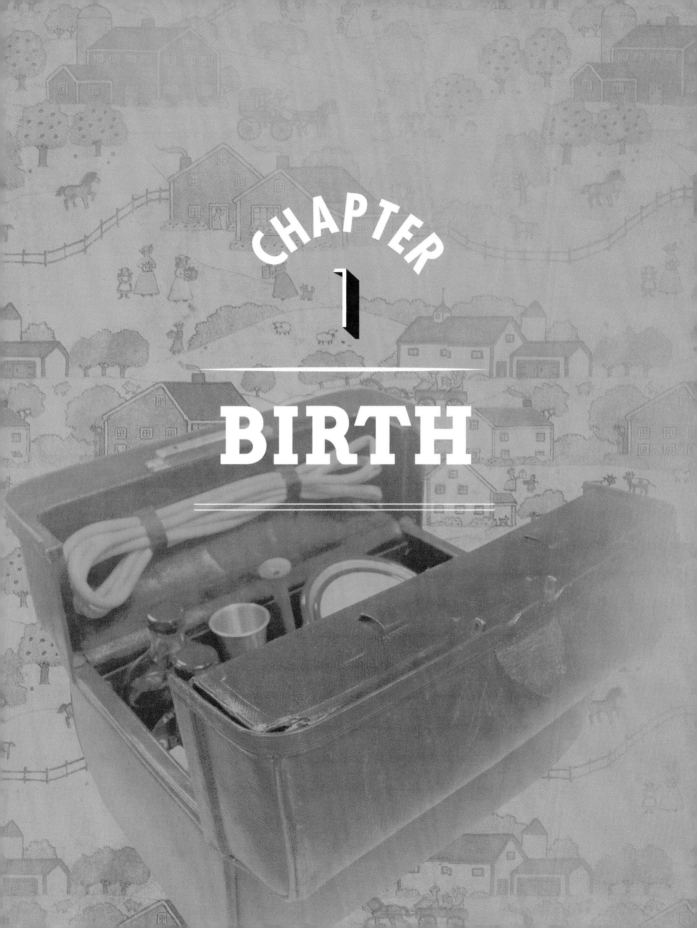

CHAPTER 1

BIRTH

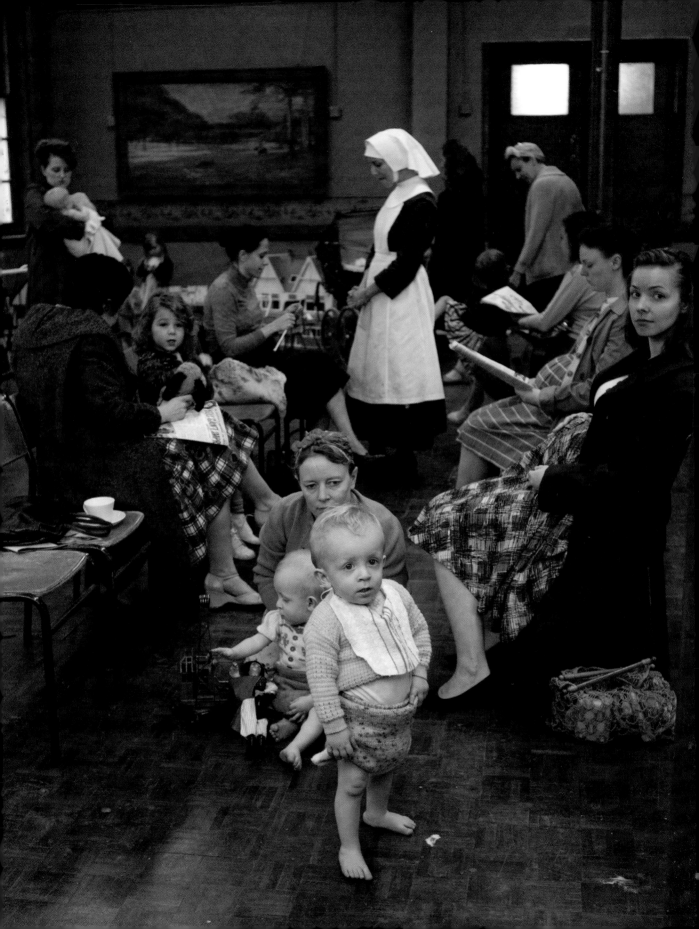

BIRTH

Everybody has a birth story, whether it is known to them or not. I was – by coincidence – brought into the world by nuns, in a small private hospital in Liverpool. The delivery was notable only for its speed. But whenever a woman visits a newly delivered relative or friend, the talk swiftly shifts from the baby to the labour: 'How was it?' we whisper. And the details are divulged and sympathised with – and will be told, and told again, in years to come. Tales such as these – ordinary, homespun, heartfelt – are the lifeblood of every *Call the Midwife* episode. And that is as it should be, for each arrival in this world is totally enthralling, a repeat beat of the greatest story ever told.

Many of the births we feature are unusual by definition. In the first series, for example, we saw the birth of triplets to an unmarried mother living in a derelict flat. Lacking even a blanket for the third child, Chummy, played by Miranda Hart, stripped down to her petticoat and wrapped him in her nurse's uniform. In another episode, she carried out a breech delivery alone, coaxing a petrified mother through the slow, controlled descent of the infant's feet and legs.

But we wanted our first birth to be an ordinary one – raw, uncomplicated, intimate, exhilarating. We wanted the fifties' trappings of the enema and shave, and the regulation left-hand-side delivery position. Above all else, however, we wanted to make it timeless, immediate and real. And so, in the opening episode of the series, ordinary unexceptional Muriel, attended by her mother, Sister Evangelina and newcomer Jenny Lee, gave birth to a boy without any complications or much fuss. It was a birth like hundreds of thousands before it, and hundreds of thousands to come – and therein lies its power.

As Pippa Harris, executive producer of *Call the Midwife*, comments, 'There is something completely universal about birth; it touches us all. You don't have to be a mother or even a woman to engage with it. All humans are drawn to it, time and again.' Mulling over the huge success of the series, she adds, 'The stakes are just so high; at any point the outcome can switch from one of joy to terrible sadness. Birth is inherently dramatic.'

No one who works on the show is more acutely tuned to the miracle of birth than Terri Coates, a midwife and lecturer of some thirty years standing. Terri, our peerless consultant midwife, has been involved with *Call the Midwife* from the start.

Terri first encountered Jennifer Worth after publishing an article in a midwifery magazine a dozen years ago, lamenting that midwives were 'almost invisible' in literature. 'Maybe,' wrote Terri, 'there is a midwife somewhere who can do for midwifery what James Herriot did for veterinary practice?'

Among many responses, Terri received a letter from retired nurse Jennifer, who said the article had inspired her to write her memoirs. Some 18 months later, she wrote again, having completed them. Terri offered to read the manuscript and was duly sent it – to her surprise, it had been written by hand on an odd assortment of pages, which she describes as being 'rather difficult to keep in order.'

'It was a lovely story about women, and for women, and it was very powerful.' Terri suggested to Jennifer that she might be able to correct some clinical errors in the text, and Jennifer – who had practised long ago and for only seven years – accepted the offer. A long and collaborative relationship ensued and, once I began to write the series, I too turned to Terri for support.

Hailed as a 'baby whisperer' by awestruck technicians, Terri is modest about her talents.

'I don't think babies are at all fazed by being on set. If you hold a newborn confidently they tend to relax and calm down very quickly.'

In fact, Terri admits she is more likely to cry than the babies, having been routinely reduced to weeping during filming. What's more, she isn't alone.

Philippa Lowthorpe, principal director of *Call the Midwife*, confesses: 'When we filmed our first birth scene – the traumatic arrival of Conchita Warren's desperately premature baby – it was such an intense experience. The film crew, Terri and I were moved to tears.' For male and female witnesses alike, all birthing scenes have proved emotional. Philippa adds, 'I have two children myself, so I should be used to it, but there is something so powerful and profound about showing a new life coming into the world, often in difficult circumstances. And, of course, these women gave birth at home, with virtually no pain relief.'

> *'I don't think babies are at all fazed by being on set. If you hold a newborn confidently they tend to relax and calm down very quickly.'*
>
> **TERRI COATES**
> *Consultant Midwife*

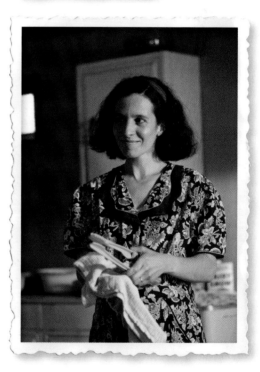

In Episode One, Jenny is given her first case to handle alone: Conchita Warren – played by Carolina Validés – who is pregnant with her 25th child.

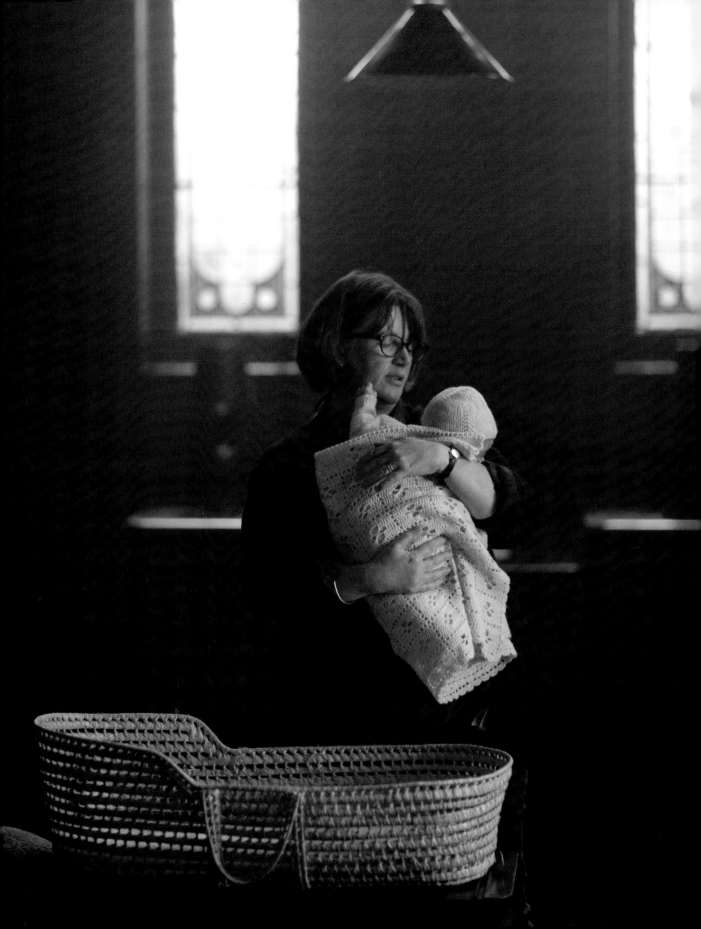

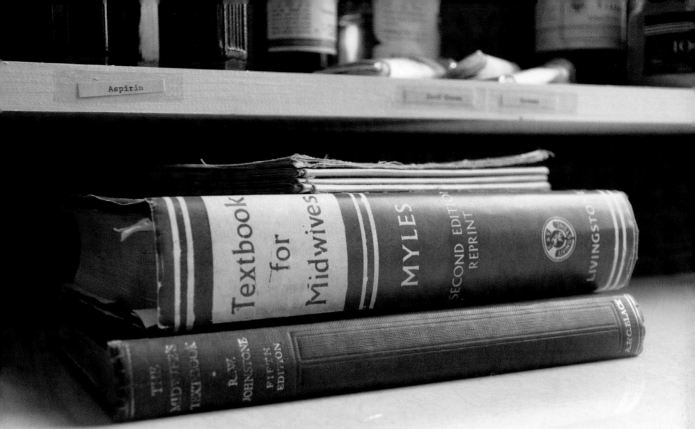

Sometimes it seems the only people on set who aren't crying in the birth scenes are the babies. Tenderly nursed by Terri, and with everyone walking on tiptoe, they often sleep deeply throughout their time on camera – which isn't necessarily what the script requires!

In real life most healthy babies are wakeful at the point of birth, and it's great to capture open eyes and flailing, starfish hands. However, we would never, ever do anything to unsettle a contented babe and the crew are adept at working round unscheduled naps. Terri occasionally sanctions gently blowing on a dozing baby's cheek, or softly tickling their feet, but if this doesn't work shots are angled so the face cannot be seen. The sound of crying – carefully recorded when it spontaneously occurs – can then be dubbed on afterwards. In addition, I usually have some emergency dialogue scribbled down

so that if I am phoned from the set with the panicky message, 'It's absolutely FAST asleep!', I can supply one of the adult actors with some explanatory lines.

Newborn babies tend not to be on the books of modelling agencies, so we recruit them direct from the maternity wings of local hospitals. During the first series, *Call the Midwife* was unknown to the masses, and we sometimes struggled to explain what we were up to. Second time around we have been bombarded, with some expectant mothers calling us direct and e-mailing photographs. Nobody has actually sent us their scan pictures yet, but it's only a matter of time.

The younger the infant, the better. In an ideal world, our babies would not be more than four days old, when they still have the glazed and curled-up look of the newly born. However, they must be licensed by their local council before

Terri Coates, Consultant Midwife,
on set tending to a newborn.

they can appear on screen, and this protective procedure takes at least a week. Second assistant director, Ben Rogers, and his team try to get one step ahead by booking babies in advance of their due date, but Mother Nature has no respect for filming schedules. We are often undone by them arriving early or too late.

Despite the nightmarish booking process, the presence of a baby brings about a tingling hush that makes the day's work special. As Pam Ferris, who plays Sister Evangelina, observes, 'It changes the atmosphere completely, you can sense something extraordinary in the air.'

Babies can 'work' for no more than twenty minutes at a time. There is more leeway with twins, who can be used alternately, but these are seldom available to us. Terri

ensures that the tiny stars are held properly, kept warm and that the surroundings are clean and hazard free. She is often contorted – out of sight of the cameras – beneath or behind the bed so as to stay within instant reach of the baby.

Natalie Hannington signed up her tiny daughter Santana – her sixth child – after seeing one of our leaflets in her maternity clinic. An eight-pound baby, Santana arrived via Caesarean section. Natalie, who is 31, describes her as 'just perfect', and was happy to share her baby with the nation on the screen.

Before appearing on camera Santana, like all performers, made a visit to make-up. There,

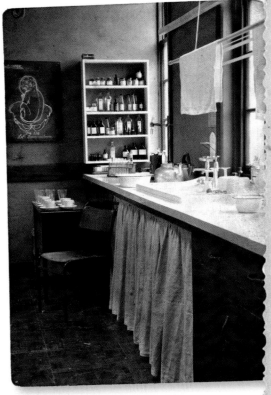

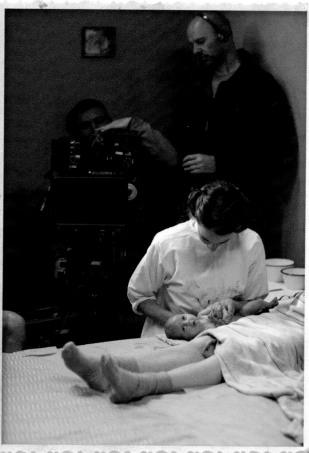

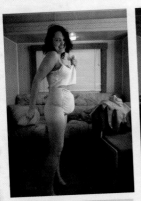
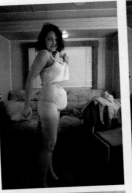
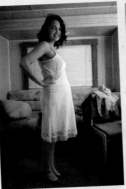
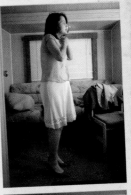
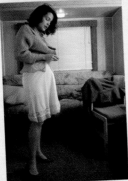
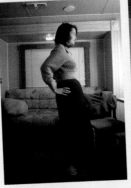
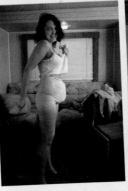
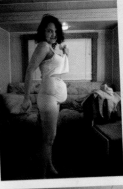
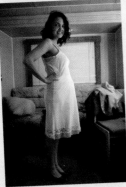
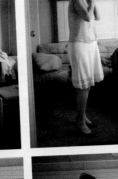
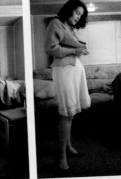
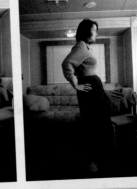
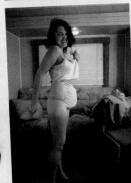
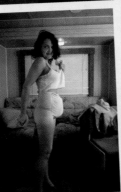
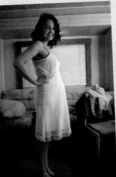
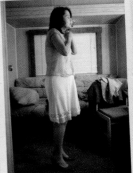

Amy Roberts, Costume Designer, has a range of pregnancy padding to hand, which actors delight in trying on.

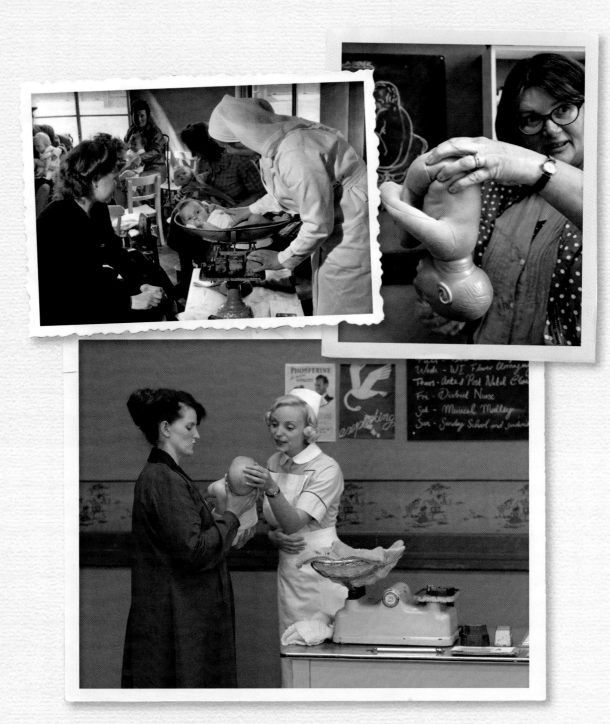

Top right: Terri Coates, Consultant Midwife, demonstrating delivery moves.
Below: Helen George (Trixie) at the maternity clinic.

she was massaged with pure grapeseed oil and 'bloodied' with a sugar-based red colouring so that she looked fresh from the womb. Many babies are also born with a coating of vernix – the white fatty substance that protects their skin in utero – and if this is required, a paste of Sudocreme and oil is carefully applied.

Christine Walmesley-Cotham, hair and make-up designer, supervises all of these preparations. Responsible for many blood-and-gore effects across the series, she is deeply involved in making pregnancy and birth look real on camera.

Christine says she is grateful that, since the advent of silicone, medical prosthetics are of a universally high quality. This lightweight malleable material offers a durability and level of detail that was not possible with latex. Silicone is used to create bumps for 'mums-to-be', which can be padded to suit the stage of a fictional pregnancy, and coloured to match the skin tone of the actress. My own favourite prostheses, however, are the exquisitely delicate umbilical cords – small coiled masterpieces of palest mauve. It seems at

once odd and entirely right that they should be kept in the make-up store, alongside the lipsticks and lacquer. For these are props from the world of women, things that are stored in the vault of all we share.

When it was time to film Santana's scene, real-life mum Natalie watched proceedings on a monitor. The baby murmured only briefly, when she was first carried into the bright light of the set, but settled within moments. Helen George, who plays Trixie, handed her to the actress playing her mother, who cradled her lovingly, and after Philippa called 'Cut!' there was the usual sound of all the male technicians clearing their throats and blowing their noses.

'It was weird to see her handed to someone else,' admits Natalie. 'But it's lovely just looking at her. It would have been fantastic to have done the same with all the other children,' she says. Like every mother who has taken part in the show, she will keep a recording of Santana's TV debut for the young star to see when she is older.

While Terri's first concern on set is always for the wellbeing of the baby, her presence is vital to the adult actors too. Some weeks before a birthing scene is filmed, the script is

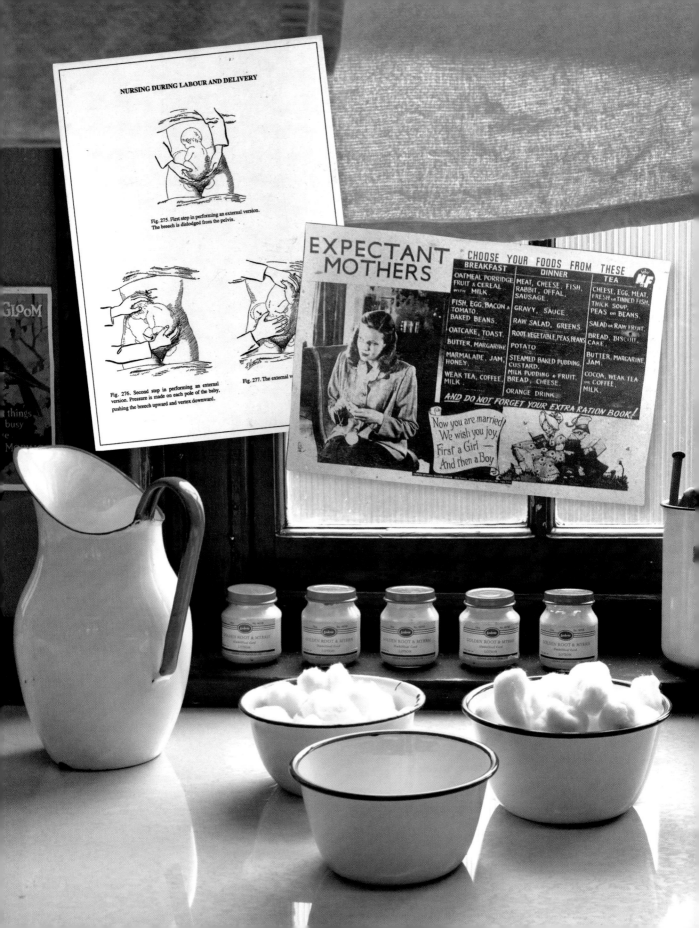

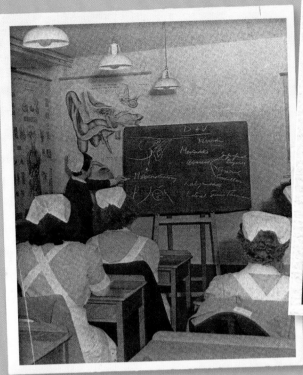

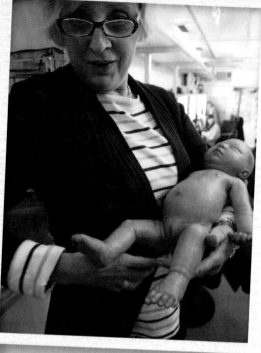

Christine Walmesley-Cotham, Hair and Make-up Designer, with one of the life-like prosthetic babies.

rehearsed in detail. Terri uses a wonderful old shabby-chic doll, which she has had throughout her career, to demonstrate the delivery moves to the actors. This is especially important when the birth is complicated. She is also careful to point out how the mother's modesty would have been preserved, and to explain key clinical phrases so that the nuns, midwives and doctors can say them with an air of confidence. She also provides crucial guidance to the actresses playing the labouring mothers. In the fifties, girls married and gave birth young, and this is reflected in the age of our performers. Very few have given birth in real life and they rely on Terri to ensure that their on-screen labour is as life-like as possible.

Terri believes that too many on-screen births are melodramatic and overly vocal. 'A lot of women are centred and calm in labour, not at all like you see in soap operas. They are focused and often very wrapped up in themselves,'

she explains. In the opinion of Pam Ferris, this approach is key to the success of the birth scenes in *Call the Midwife*. 'We've had fabulous actresses doing the birthing, making really believable noises. The emotional temperature in the room is really high when we're doing those sequences,' says Pam. 'It's very, very powerful stuff. You don't get much more fundamental than that really. The anxiety and the joy combined make them very, very highly charged moments for everybody. Although we're sometimes only giving birth to a little bit of plastic, you still get excited.'

These 'little bits of plastic' are actually prosthetic babies, which appear in almost every episode. They take the place of real babies in the more technically complex delivery shots.

The detailed small figures have the dimensions of a six-and-a-half-pound infant, but weigh rather more, and have a wipe-clean silicone skin that can be dressed with oils, gels and creams.

THE MEDICAL BAG

BEING A FIFTIES' MIDWIFE REQUIRED COMPASSION, MEDICAL KNOW-HOW AND MUSCLE-POWER. THE BROWN LEATHER CASE TAKEN TO EVERY DELIVERY BY THE MIDWIVES WEIGHED AT LEAST AS MUCH AS A LUSTY NEWBORN. SO WHAT WAS INSIDE WEIGHING IT DOWN?

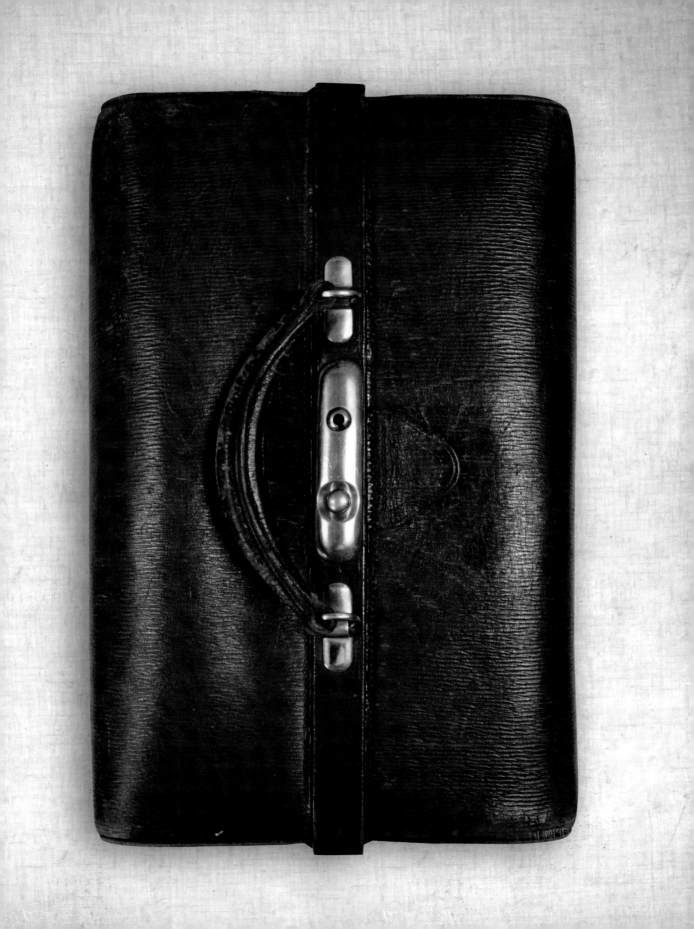

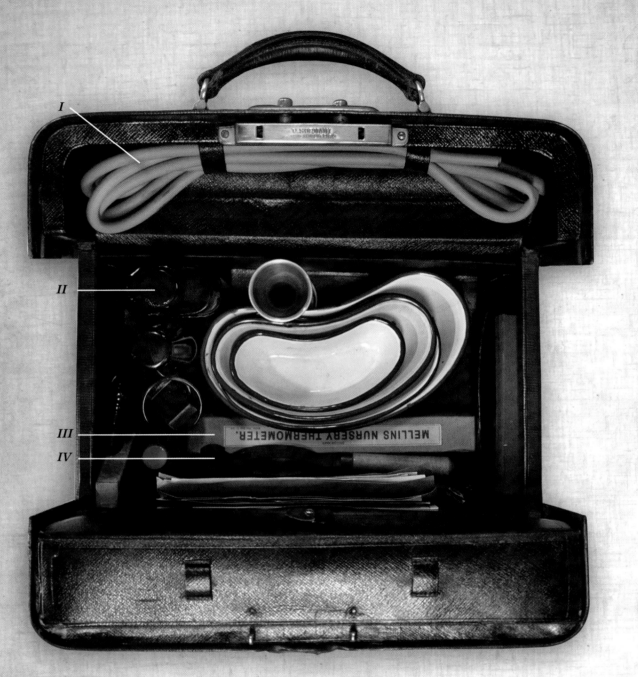

FIGURE 1 – OPEN MIDWIFE'S MEDICAL BAG

I. There was a length of rubber tubing with which to give an enema. At the time the midwives and nuns were switching from old-style and easily smashed glass to rubber. Back then every woman in labour was given an enema but they are no longer deemed necessary during childbirth. — *II.* Dettol was a well-known antiseptic. Today its function has largely been replaced by plain water after fears that strong antiseptics kill good bacteria as well as bad. — *III.* There was a nursery thermometer for testing bath water – now mostly usurped by an elbow or a wrist – as well as one to register body temperature. — *IV.* The urine in a test tube held by clamps was warmed to see if there was any evidence of protein. If the heated urine produced a frothy substance resembling cooked egg white then it indicated a possible infection or even the threat of pre-eclampsia, a condition that can be fatal to mums and babies. Nowadays strips are used to carry out the same test. A spirit lamp – a bottle with a wick running through it – was lit for urine testing, which explains why midwives carried a box of matches with them.

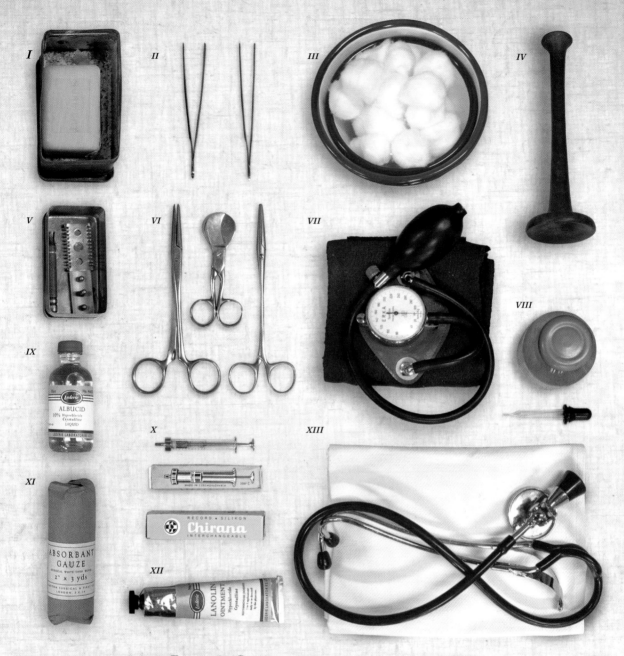

FIGURE 2 – CONTENTS OF A MIDWIFE'S MEDICAL BAG

I. Carbolic soap helped the shaving process, and was also used for handwashing. — *II.* Tweezers were used to remove dirty dressings, which were duly dropped into an enamel bowl. — *III.* Enamel bowls were carried to hold solutions or waste items. — *IV.* The horn-shaped Pinard, a foetal heart monitor, has been standard equipment for decades. — *V.* A vicious-looking stainless steel razor was used to prepare women for delivery. — *VI.* Scissors used to cut the umbilical cord are shaped like a parrot's beak. — *VII.* Midwives carried a sphygmomanometer or blood pressure measuring device with a fabric cuff and the dial encased in leather. — *VIII.* This hypochlorite solution was used as a steriliser. — *IX.* This ergometrine oxytocic was injected to stop bleeding after childbirth by encouraging the uterus to contract. — *X.* Syringes were used to administer the ergometrine. — *XI.* Gauze was used to tie off the umbilical cord. It was replaced first by rubber bands and then by plastic clips. — *XII.* Midwives carried a tube of Lanolin for women preparing to breastfeed, to prevent sore nipples. — *XIII.* A stethoscope – invented in France at the beginning of the 19th century.

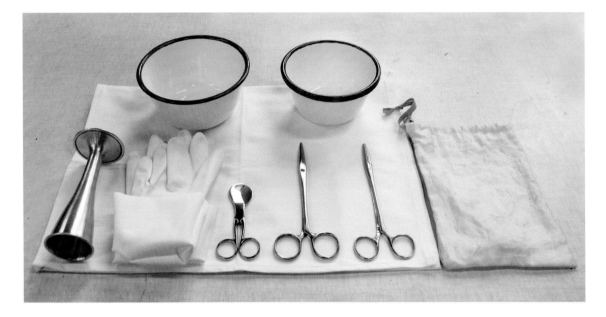

The midwives would unpack and lay out essential items such as scissors, bowls and gloves, on a chest of drawers or bedside table, within arm's reach.

The oils, gels and creams are used to match the actual babies used in close-ups. Disconcertingly, the prosthetic babies have interchangeable male and female genitalia, though these are never seen. Robust enough for repeated, long-term use, the handmade dolls cost £5,000 apiece and are treated with the utmost care.

Terri's expertise provides an essential link between past and present on the show. Having qualified in 1982, she worked alongside many midwives who would have been Jenny Lee's contemporaries. From them, she learned about the methods in use decades previously. Perhaps surprisingly, relatively little has altered.

'Babies still come out in exactly the same way,' smiles Terri, mulling over the small but distinct changes in practice that have occurred down the years. 'For example, in the fifties, midwives always wore masks. It isn't that long ago we stopped wearing them, but we don't use them in the show because masks don't make for good television!' She adds, 'Although we probably have more disposable items now, much of the equipment is largely the same.'

Terri herself still uses the same wooden Pinard – a horn-shaped foetal heart monitor – she bought when she first qualified as a midwife thirty years ago.

Some aspects of childbirth have changed beyond all recognition. As Terri says, 'Women in the fifties expected to give birth at home, with only very basic pain relief, and as a result they coped.'

In fact, in Series One of *Call the Midwife*, the women were offered no help with pain at all.

Pam Ferris (Sister Evangelina) and Jessica Raine (Jenny) with Emma Noakes, who played Shirley Redmond in Episode Four.

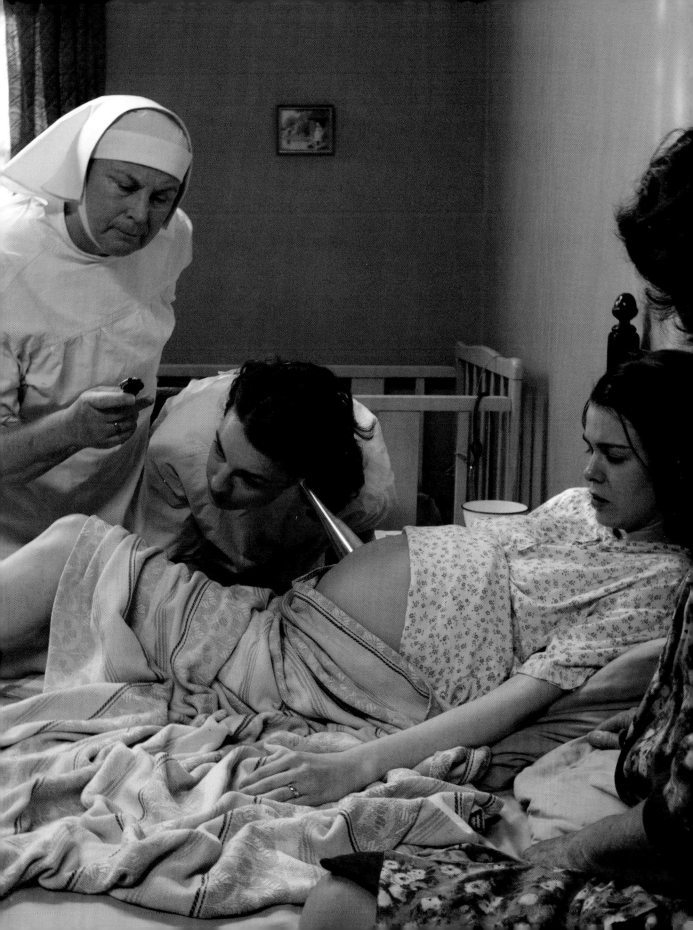

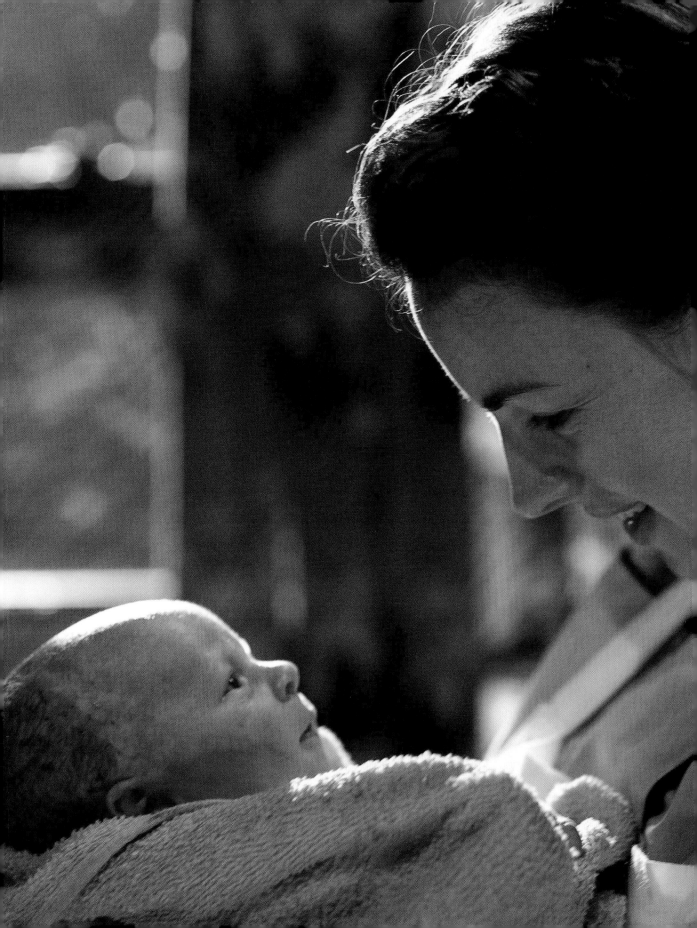

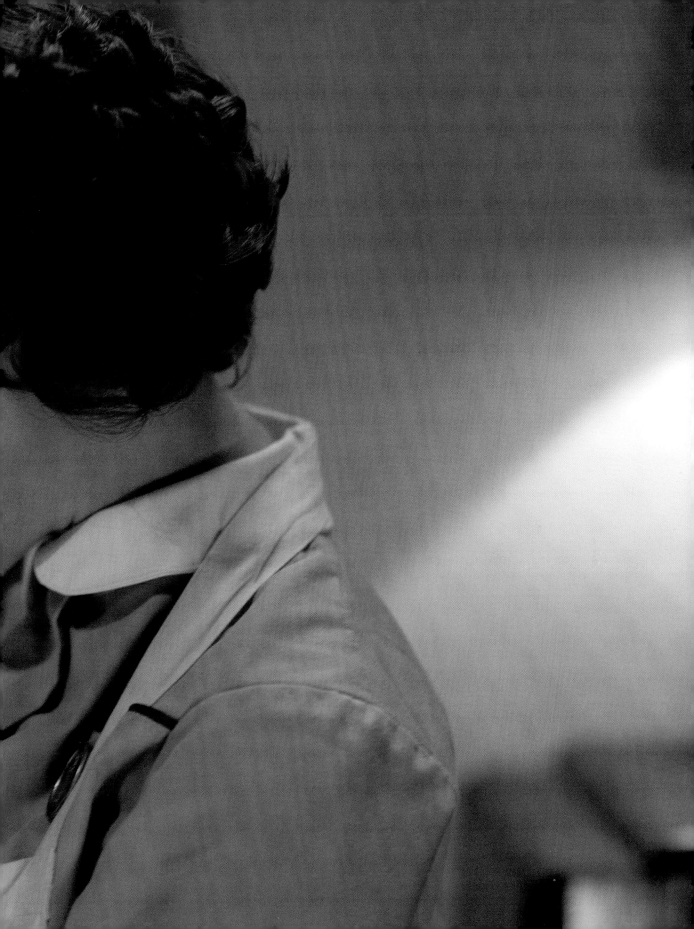

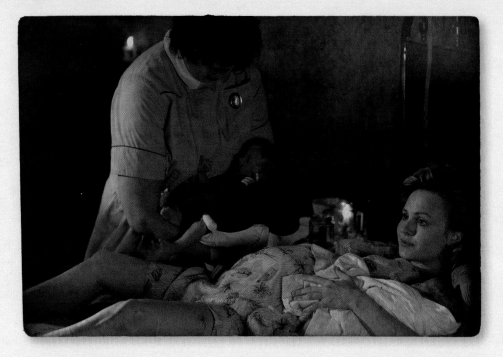

Miranda Hart (Chummy Browne) and Tina O'Brien, who played Cathy Powell in Episode Six.

I had queried this with Jennifer Worth, after reading the original books. She replied that it had been impossible for the midwives to transport cylinders of gas-and-air on their bicycles. Even the 'portable' units were packed into heavy cases, and the only space on the bike was taken by the midwife's bag.

Further research revealed that in the fifties a furore was brewing regarding pain relief in labour – almost one hundred years after it was introduced. The numbing qualities of ether and chloroform (chemicals that had to be inhaled) were discovered in the middle of the 19th century. They were swiftly pressed into use for all types of surgery, and it wasn't long before their potential for use in childbirth was spotted.

The first woman anaesthetised during labour in the United States was Fanny Longfellow, the wife of poet and abolitionist Henry, in 1847. She later called ether 'the greatest blessing of our age'. Meanwhile, in England, the anaesthetic power of chloroform found an illustrious fan. Queen Victoria enjoyed a happy marriage to Prince Albert, but it came at a high price – one pregnancy after another. Her labours were torture to her, and indeed she suffered so greatly that when her eldest child, the Crown Princess of Prussia, wrote to say she was expecting her own first baby, the Queen wrote back offering not congratulations but the tart comment, 'This is HORRID news.'

The Queen's doctors debated the value of pain relief at length before deciding to use it for her eighth delivery. Her Majesty gave birth to Prince Leopold George Duncan Albert on 7 April 1853, after inhaling chloroform from a handkerchief for 52 minutes. She described the relief this gave her as 'delightful beyond measure', and allowed her use of anaesthesia to be made public. Thereafter, this particular method was known as 'Chloroform à La Reine'.

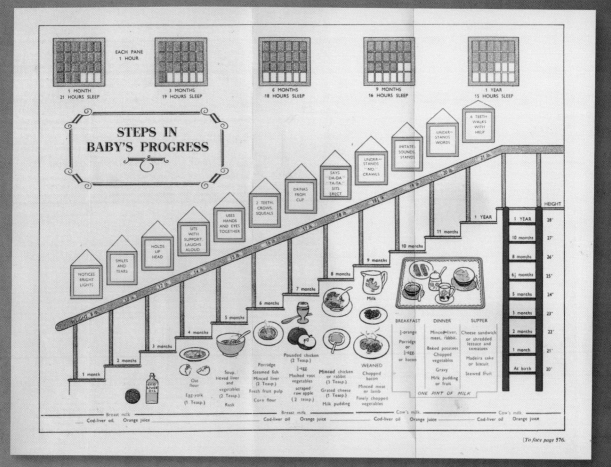

STEPS IN BABY'S PROGRESS

EACH PANE 1 HOUR

1 MONTH — 21 HOURS SLEEP
3 MONTHS — 19 HOURS SLEEP
6 MONTHS — 18 HOURS SLEEP
9 MONTHS — 16 HOURS SLEEP
1 YEAR — 15 HOURS SLEEP

NOTICES BRIGHT LIGHTS
SMILES AND TEARS
HOLDS UP HEAD
SITS WITH SUPPORT. LAUGHS ALOUD
USES HANDS AND EYES TOGETHER
2 TEETH. CROWS. SQUEALS
DRINKS FROM CUP
SAYS "DA-DA" "TA-TA." SITS ERECT
UNDERSTANDS "NO." CRAWLS
IMITATES SOUNDS. STANDS
UNDERSTANDS WORDS
6 TEETH. WALKS WITH HELP

WEIGHT 8 lb. — 10 lb. — 12 lb. — 14 lb. — 15 lb. — 16 lb. — 17 lb. — 18 lb. — 18½ lb. — 19 lb. — 20 lb. — 21 lb.

1 month — 2 months — 3 months — 4 months — 5 months — 6 months — 7 months — 8 months — 9 months — 10 months — 11 months — 1 YEAR

HEIGHT

1 YEAR	28"
10 months	27"
8 months	26"
6½ months	25"
5 months	24"
3 months	23"
2 months	22"
1 month	21"
At birth	20"

Oat flour
Egg-yolk (1 Teasp.)

Soup, sieved liver and vegetables (2 Teasp.)
Rusk

Porridge
Steamed fish
Minced liver (2 Teasp.)
Fresh fruit pulp
Corn flour

Pounded chicken (2 Teasp.)
½-egg
Mashed root vegetables
scraped raw apple (2 teasp.)

Minced chicken or rabbit (3 Teasp.)
Grated cheese (1 Teasp.)
Milk pudding

WEANED
Chopped bacon
Minced meat or lamb
Finely chopped vegetables

Milk

BREAKFAST	DINNER	SUPPER
½-orange	Minced liver, meat, rabbit.	Cheese sandwich or shredded lettuce and tomatoes
Porridge or ½-egg or bacon	Baked potatoes	
	Chopped vegetables	Madeira cake or biscuit
	Gravy	Stewed fruit
	Milk pudding or fruit	

ONE PINT OF MILK

Breast milk ————— Cod-liver oil — Orange juice ————— Breast milk — Cod-liver oil — Orange juice ————— Cow's milk — Cod-liver oil — Orange juice ————— Cow's milk — Cod-liver oil — Orange juice

(To face page 576.

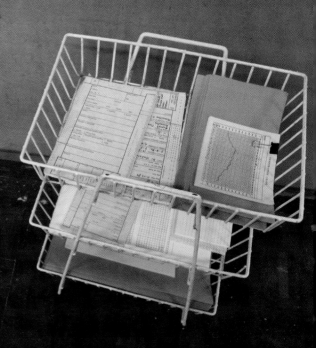

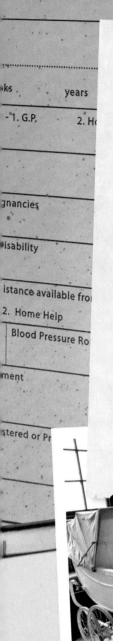

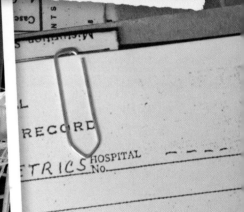

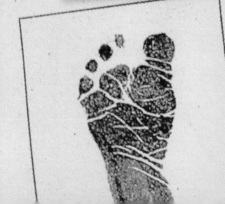

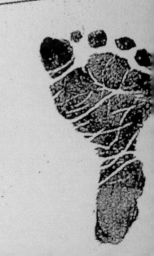

By the fifties ether and chloroform had been replaced by Trilene and gas-and-air, which was inhaled during contractions through special apparatus. Trilene, which was blue, smelled like dry-cleaning fluid. However, the kit it required was relatively light, and the assumption was that bicycle-riding midwives could transport it easily.

At the end of 1955, 259 Trilene sets were in use in the UK, and by the end of 1956 this had risen to roughly 900 sets. In 1957, an estimated 1,259 sets were being pedalled around the country by district midwives. Unfortunately, that still only represented one set of equipment for every six midwives. This caused such anger that questions were asked in Parliament – the inhalers were simply not being manufactured in sufficient numbers.

Gas-and-air, which both mothers and midwives preferred, remained too cumbersome for transportation by bike. In Parliament in 1959, the Minister of Health was quizzed by the MP representing Stoke-on-Trent. When, he demanded, was the Government going to provide midwives with motor vehicles so that they could transport gas-and-air to their patients? The Minister for Health sidestepped this rather nimbly, saying it was a 'question for the local authorities'.

Pain relief was, of course, available in hospitals and in the small GP-led units on offer in certain areas. Very slowly, the tide began to turn against home births. In the minds of many women, a hospital birth meant a safe birth. For countless generations, being 'brought to bed' had been such a risky business that the church offered a special service called the Thanksgiving For Women After Childbirth in which mothers could kneel at the altar and give thanks for their survival.

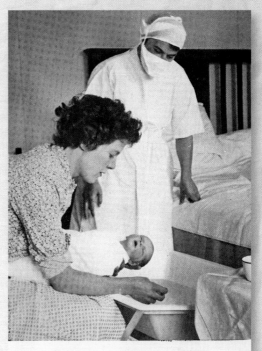

The midwife helps and encourages the young mother as she learns to bath her baby

Even in the fifties, as in the present day, there were some complications that could not be overcome. The first series of *Call the Midwife* includes one of the saddest stories from the books, that of the young and beautiful Margaret Jones, recently married to a man rather older than herself. At the happiest point of their life together, she collapses with eclampsia, an acute complication of pregnancy. Despite the emergency delivery of her stillborn premature daughter – the only cure for the condition – Margaret dies, leaving her husband bereft. Margaret's illness was sudden and severe. Had symptoms developed more slowly, the threat to her life might have been diagnosed and averted. In almost every episode of *Call the*

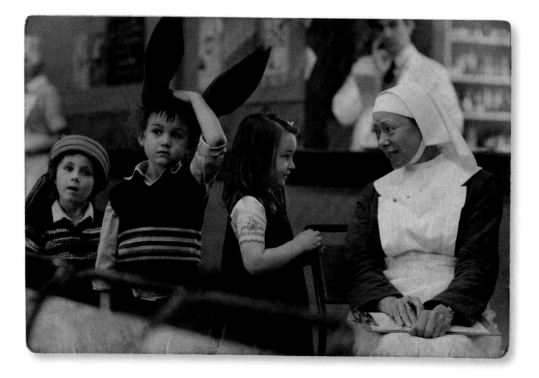

Midwife, we see the midwives boiling urine in test tubes over spirit lamps: it was to test for the presence of protein in the water. Along with high blood pressure and fluid retention, protein in the urine indicates pre-eclampsia. In the fifties, medical professionals believed that the condition could be held at bay with bed-rest, sedation and a special diet. Today, drugs are used to help control the blood pressure, and the baby's condition is carefully monitored. The mother can survive, and her baby be safely delivered.

A 1959 government enquiry into maternity services carefully weighed up the pros and cons of home versus hospital deliveries, but was uncompromising in its admiration of one thing: midwives. It remarked, 'The midwife's three assets of time, skill and attitude of mind are of immense value to her patient,' but was also forced to state, 'Even if the financial resources were available to provide hospital beds for all confinements there would appear to be little prospect of finding enough midwives to staff them.'

More than sixty years on, it seems not much has changed. In July 2012, 25 midwifery students – dressed like Chummy and Jenny in blue dresses and red cardigans – rode vintage bikes to the Houses of Parliament. There, they served cake to MPs in a bid to persuade them to invest in training midwives. There are, insist the students, not enough to go around.

As they cycled through Westminster shouting, 'Call for more midwives!' I felt utterly humbled by their passion for their craft. For this is what midwives do – they live and breathe the beauty of their calling. It inspires and sustains them, just as they inspire and sustain the women they support.

The rewards of their vocation are life-long. Terri once said, 'Birth amazes me. And if it ever stops amazing me then I will know it is time to give up and get out of the profession. I'm still awed by every birth I attend.'

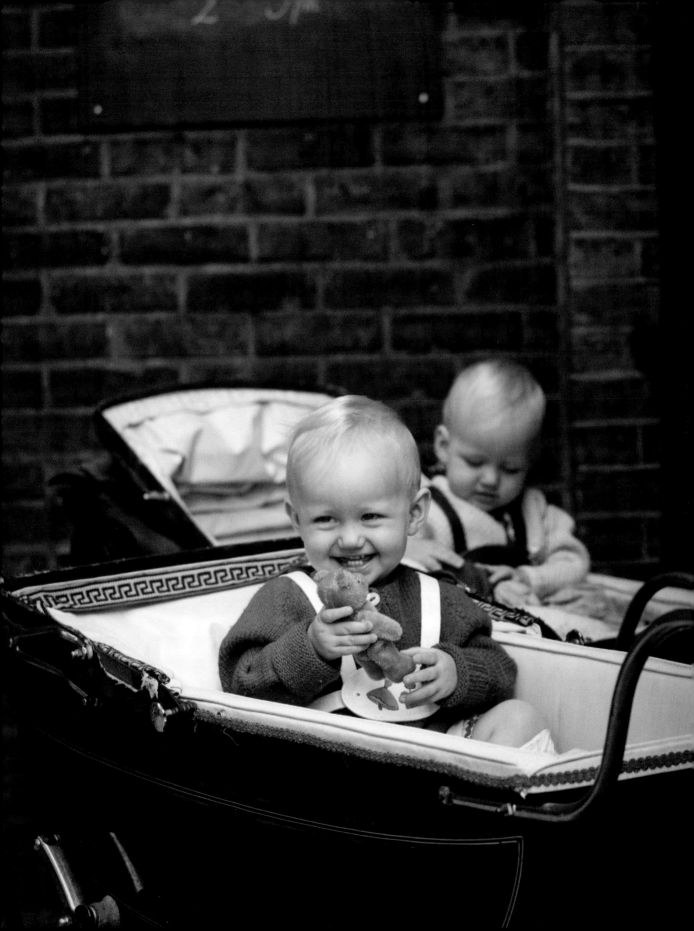

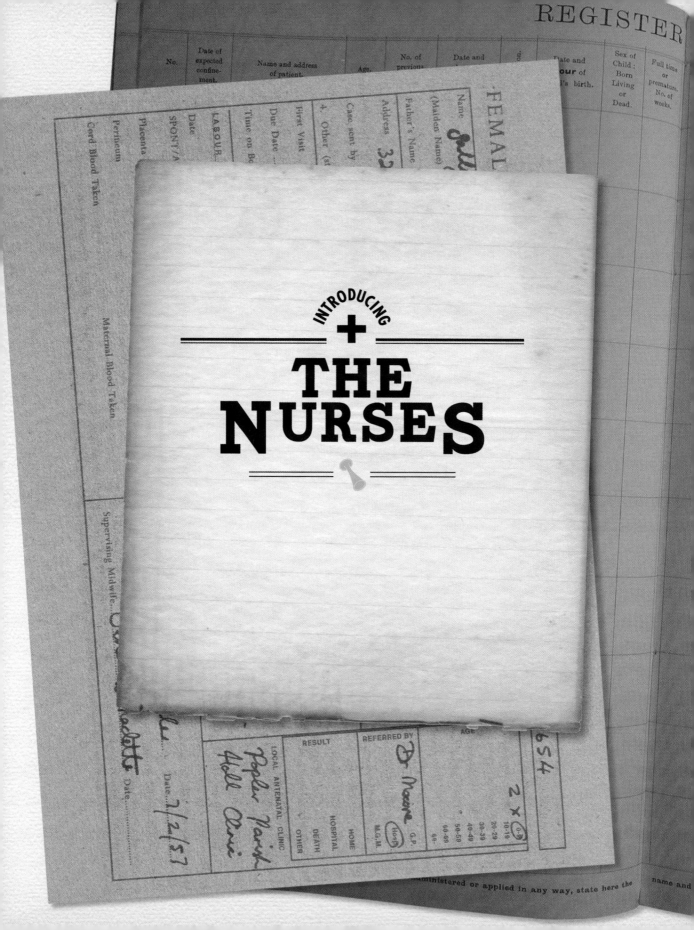

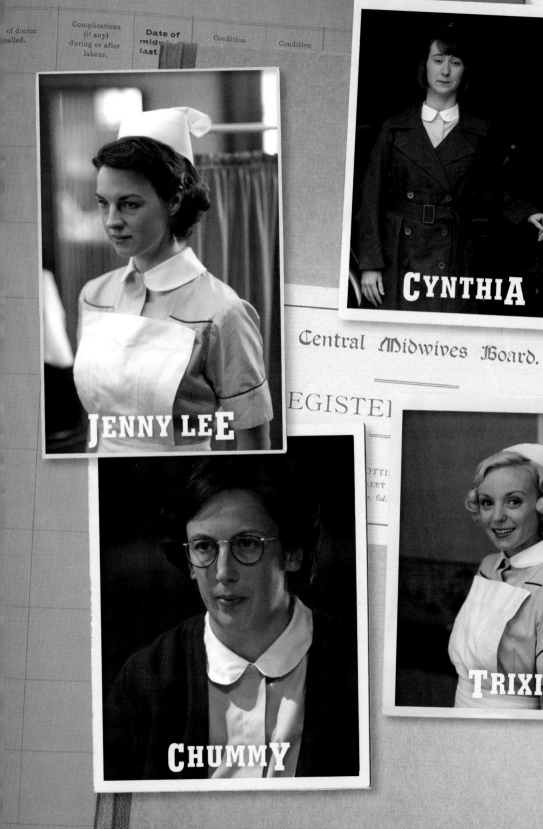

CASES.

of doctor called.	Complications (if any) during or after labour.	Date of mid... last	Condition	Condition

JENNY LEE

CYNTHIA

Central Midwives Board.

EGISTE

CHUMMY

TRIXIE

PROFILE + JENNY

Jennifer Worth expressed very little interest in who would eventually play her. When we used to play at putting an imaginary cast together, she would change the subject when it came to the character of Jenny. Apart from expressing an entirely natural desire that the girl we hired should be good looking, she claimed to have no opinion at all. She didn't fictionalise 'Jenny Lee' in her *Call the Midwife* books – she used her own name, and set herself upon the page quite plainly. I often wondered if she regretted this.

What Jennifer was always very clear about, however, was that she would like the series to give young, unknown performers a chance to shine. Our casting director, Andy Pryor, is a tremendous spotter of new talent, and his first trawl of 'Jennys' was fantastic. Most of them were unknown to me and I knew this would please

Jennifer. By this stage, she was acutely ill and, although I knew we couldn't rush the process, I was desperate to cast the part before she died. For all she feigned indifference, I had a gut feeling that she actually DID want to know who was going to play the part.

Every girl who auditioned for the part had something brilliant to commend her, but a lot of them were just a bit too modern. But then I saw Jessica Raine's audition tape and suddenly sat up straight. Here was someone with cut-glass pronunciation that didn't sound like a parody, and an inner strength that didn't seem too bold: Jessica Raine. She had come close to being overlooked, but was invited to the next round of auditions and Philippa Lowthorpe, the director, e-mailed me excitedly: 'We got Jessica back – she was fantastic!!' That was it – we offered her the job.

With the success of the first series, Jessica became a star overnight. But no success – especially in show business – is ever truly instant. Like many a performer, she worked long and hard to achieve her aims.

Jessica grew up on a farm in rural Herefordshire. Her heart was set on acting from childhood. 'I knew I wanted to act but I didn't say so for years, because it seemed unattainable as a career,' she reveals.

'I did A level Theatre Studies and had an incredibly inspirational teacher. That's what makes teaching so vital. He touched a lot of people's lives.'

Jessica went on to study drama at University of the West of England, then waitressed while seeking roles in local plays. It strikes me that Jennifer would have had every sympathy with Jessica's early deliberations, for she too took time to find her feet professionally. Leaving school in her mid-teens, she learned shorthand and typing, working in a boys' grammar school before applying to train as a nurse.

Jessica's path to drama school in the capital was similarly vexed, but, like the woman she went on to immortalise on screen, she refused to be daunted. Despite being turned down by RADA, she moved to London and worked in a call centre while building up to having another go. Further rejections from other drama schools followed, but she persisted and applied to RADA once again. This time, she succeeded.

'By this time I felt there was no possibility I was going to get in, but there was nothing to lose. And as soon as I relaxed and stopped trying to impress people, the real me came out. That was a lesson for life.'

After graduating from RADA, Jessica appeared in a number of National Theatre

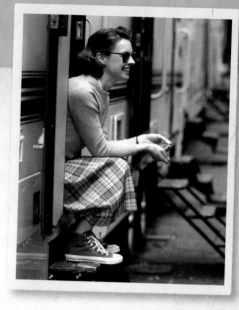

productions, often playing angry young women with a lot to say. 'I got a lot off my chest when I was doing that!' she laughs.

Jessica finds a great deal to interest her in the role of Jenny, who is so different to the rebellious youngsters she has previously played. 'She has so much empathy, she is young, not particularly innocent, but she looks at things with such new eyes.'

Jessica is in awe of what young midwives such as Jenny, Trixie and Cynthia accomplished in the course of their daily work. 'It is that sense of command and calm that is really important. You have got to be in control; you are dealing with a woman going through a lot of pain and she could be really terrified.'

By the time Jessica was cast, Jennifer was too ill to meet her. However we were able to show her photographs. She looked at the pictures of the young actress for a long time, stroking the black and white shadows on the paper. And she pronounced herself satisfied. That was all that mattered.

Jessica Raine and I picked up our scripts and set off into the future.

Q&A

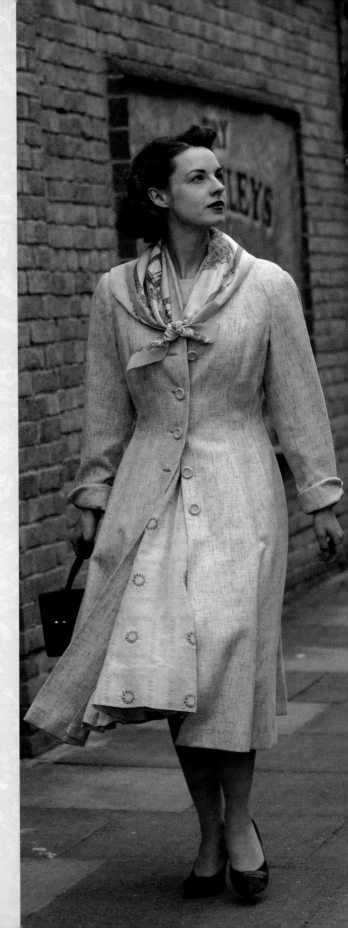

What is your favourite outfit?
A cream New Look style coat I had tailor-made.
I had to save up for ages, but it was worth
the wait.

Where do you go on holiday?
I spent six months in Paris after leaving school.
I've been back three times, and never tire of it.

**Who is your dream date and where would
you go?**
I'm a classically trained pianist, so I'd love to go
back in time and meet one of the great musicians,
such as Frederic Chopin. He would give me
a piano lesson, and then we would go out to
dinner, perhaps on a mountainside, or with
a view of a lake. That would be perfect.

What is your favourite record and film?
Mario Lanza singing 'Be My Love', and 'Brief
Encounter'. They both remind me of someone
very dear to me, and a situation that we could
not change.

What is your most treasured memory?
Opening the letter telling me I had been accepted
to train as a nurse.

Your favourite meal?
Escalopes of veal, followed by Peach Melba.

What do you do in your spare time?
I'm a member of a music club, and I although
I don't drink much alcohol, I also love to visit the
pubs of the East End with my friends. The Prospect
of Whitby, down by the river, is a great favourite
with all of us.

What's your secret vice?
It's not actually that secret – bright red lipstick!

And your most shining virtue?
I never give in to tiredness.

**Where would you like to be in five years'
time?**
Making my way up the medical ladder. Perhaps
as a ward sister in a London teaching hospital.

PROFILE + CYNTHIA

Cynthia Miller and Jennifer met on the latter's first day in Poplar, and a connection evolved that lasted until Cynthia's death from cancer in 2006. Indeed, the final volume of the *Call the Midwife* trilogy, *Farewell To The East End*, carries the dedication, 'To Cynthia, for a lifetime of friendship'. Her name remained unaltered in the series, at Jennifer's insistence, and I was intrigued by their special connection, and very respectful of it. However, though Jennifer wanted Cynthia enshrined, as a memorial to the affection they had shared, she would not speak of her in any great detail. Then, on my very last visit to Jennifer, she went to great pains to get out her wedding album in order to show me a photo of her friend. It depicted Cynthia at the end of a row of guests. In a hat and belted coat, she looked shy and slightly out of things. 'She was always so very

unassuming,' sighed Jennifer, closing the album.

When I settled down to work on the character of Cynthia, I decided the best approach was to treat her as special, but not unique. The world is full of young Cynthias – shy, quiet girls who feel things deeply, yet can be funny and playful in the company of friends. Weaving the scripts, I inched forward delicately, hoping to balance respect for Cynthia's memory with the need to write a role that would interest an actor. Somewhere along the way, things must have clicked into place a little, because when Bryony Hannah read the script she wanted the job. 'I was just really delighted by it. You know when you read a character if it is something you feel you are able to do, and you just hope you are the right person for it,' she explains.

We cast Bryony without hesitation. Fresh from huge West End success in the play *The*

Children's Hour, we had no doubts about her talent, or that she could project the goodness and sincerity that Cynthia required.

'I feel Cynthia is a younger person than me, and a little more naive than I am now. Her profession is totally alien to me but she is very kind and generous. She is giving, yet there is anxiety beneath that sometimes. It makes her a more rounded character.'

In the course of the role, Bryony has become adept at handling newborns. 'The baby scenes are very humbling – you have a great responsibility, obviously,' she says. But handling the infants has stirred up deeper feelings. 'I was broody beforehand. It hasn't made it worse, but it has compounded it.'

The birth scenes are always very intense, to the point where they can take an actual, physical toll. 'It is so tense, and you get so involved,' explains Bryony. The delivery of Winnie Lawson's mixed-race baby in Series One was a case in point. 'I got to the end of it all and found I was hardly breathing.

'With my role I am trying to be as honest as I can, to allow the inner character to seep through. When playing emotional scenes I just want to be able to do the writing justice.'

Bryony first made up her mind to be an actor as a child, after watching black and white movies starring Fred Astaire and John Wayne.

'Whenever I thought I wanted to be something else, it was only ever because of a film! I thought about chasing tornadoes after seeing *Twister*. I wanted to be a marine biologist after *Free Willy*.'

Nevertheless, it took time to see that dream become reality. She worked in pubs in her home town of Portsmouth, and sought roles in fringe theatre before getting into RADA at the fourth attempt. This enforced delay rather pleases her, with hindsight.

'I don't think I could have coped at eighteen. Twenty-one, the age I finally went there, is still young. I also looked at the year groups that came before me and I knew I wouldn't have fitted in.' As it happened, she attended the school at the same time as Jessica Raine, and with the success of *Call the Midwife*, their fortunes remain entwined.

At present, Bryony's life is consumed by work, to the point where even her spare time is spent at the theatre.

'I am writing a list of exciting things to do before I'm 30,' she confides. 'But, with the exception of jet skiing it's looking woefully empty!'

One suspects that the shadowy, real-life Cynthia might have rather approved …

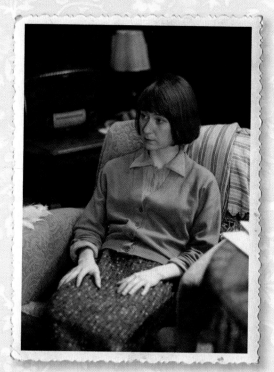

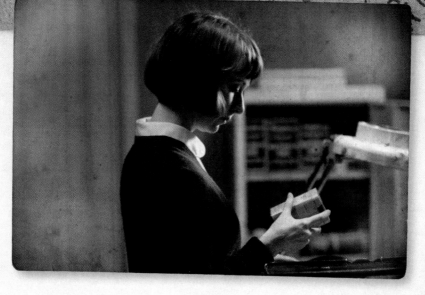

Q&A

What is your favourite outfit?
My floral dressing gown. My grandmother made it for me from a bedspread, not long after the War.

Where do you go on holiday?
I'm quite keen on Youth Hostelling, and last year I took my bike and cycled all over Derbyshire.

Who is your dream date and where would you go?
I think I'd be too nervous to enjoy an actual date, unless it was with someone I'd known for a long time. I'd quite like a penfriend – maybe someone living in America or Australia.

What is your favourite record and film?
I love the song 'I'm Always Chasing Rainbows' – it's been recorded so many times, but I never mind who's singing it. And I adored Walt Disney's *Lady and the Tramp*.

What is your most treasured memory?
As a student nurse, I looked after a little boy who was desperately ill with polio. He was in an iron lung to begin with, but eventually walked out of the hospital under his own steam. As he left, he turned round and said, 'Thank you'.

Your favourite meal?
Roast chicken, with all the trimmings. And rhubarb fool. I love rhubarb.

What do you do in your spare time?
Chummy's been teaching me how to use the sewing machine. And I help out with Girls' Brigade.

What's your secret vice?
Emergency Ward 10. I sometimes time my housecalls so that when it's on I'll be at a house with a television set. And then I look at Dr Dawson over the patient's shoulder.

And your most shining virtue?
I don't think I have one. But I try to be kind.

Where would you like to be in five years' time?
In the right place. And I'm not sure where that is yet.

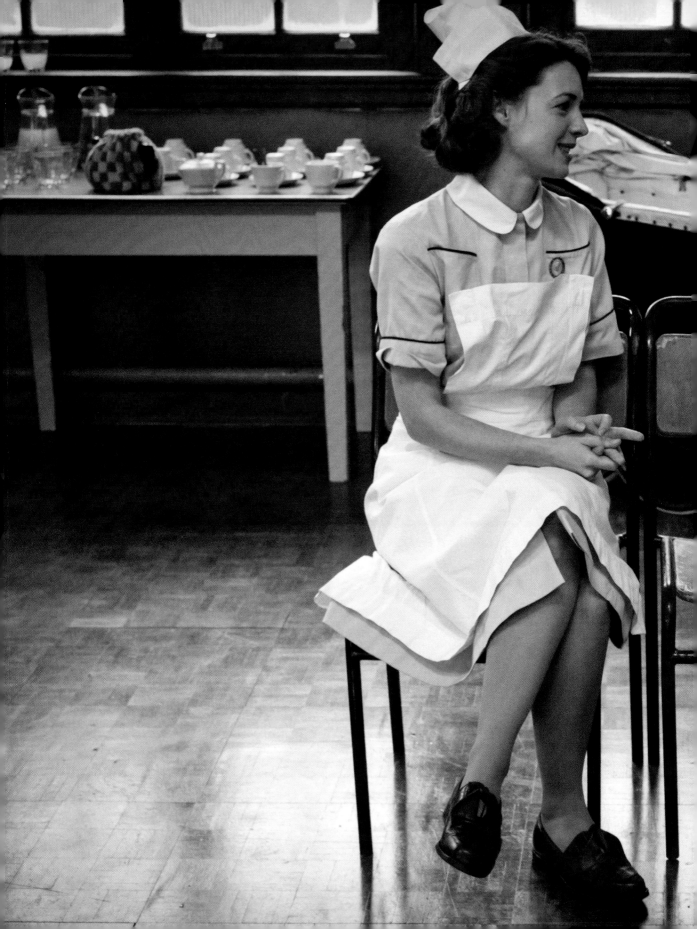

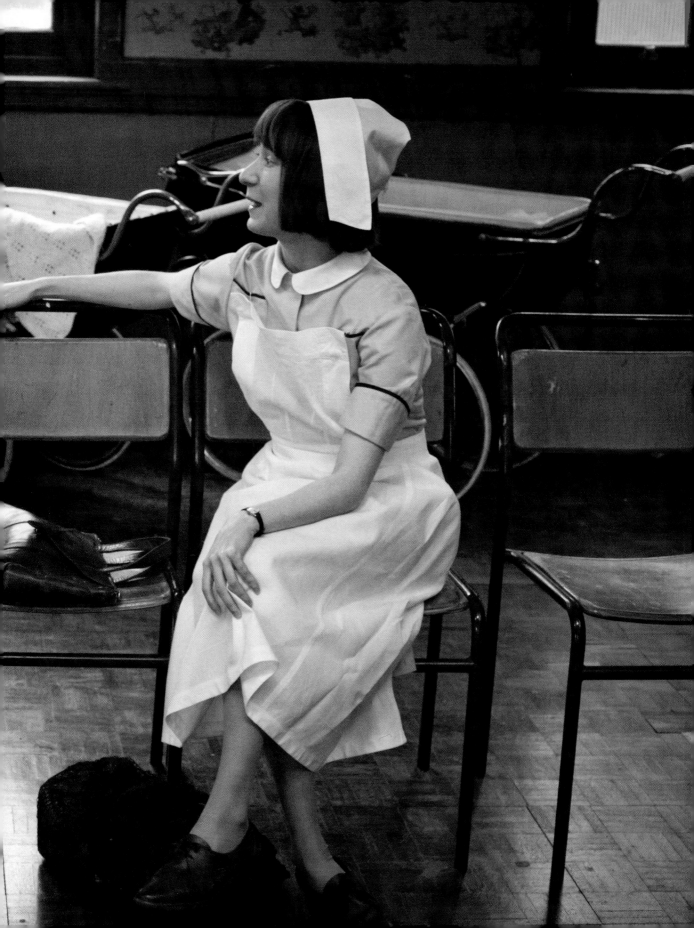

PROFILE
+
CHUMMY

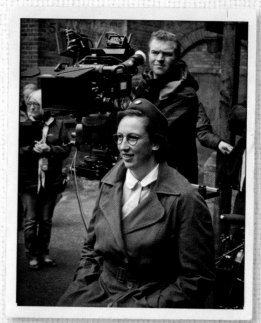

T here has been some debate as to whether 'Chummy' ever actually existed. Her full name – Camilla Fortescue-Cholmondely-Browne – seems implausible enough to be a pseudonym. In the original book, she was described as the daughter of a Governor of Rajahstan, but when the script team looked into this, it raised immediate questions. Rajahstan did not exist until after partition in 1947, whereafter all Governors were Indian. On two separate occasions, Jennifer Worth gave Pippa and I different names for her, but by then she was ill, and they did not tally. On our final visit to her she also showed us a photograph of a tall and mannish nurse, who she said was Chummy, but it passed through our hands but briefly, and the trail went cold. If Chummy is a fiction, perhaps it doesn't matter. Miranda Hart was captivated from the off.

'I was in the middle of writing my own series and I thought, "I'm too busy to read this". But after I read the first chapter I fell in love with the Chummy in the book. And when I read the scripts I thought, "These are brilliant".'

Pippa invited Miranda to lunch at Neal Street Production headquarters. As we tucked in to our sandwiches, we were told that Sam Mendes – director of the latest Bond film – was auditioning girls in the room across the corridor. Peering through the glass door, we watched them trooping in and out of his office. 'Why doesn't he ask us?' said Miranda, 'We'd be much better.' The three of us laughed a lot that day, which seemed to seal the deal – ironically, perhaps, as this would be Miranda's first straight role. She was keen to stretch herself dramatically after the success of her eponymous sitcom. Since it was first aired on TV in 2009, Miranda has won her an army of fans and a mantelshelf full of awards.

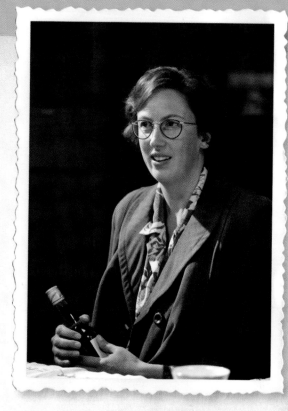

'Not having to get a laugh is a nice change,' she admits. 'Having done two series of my situation comedy, it was marvellous to do something a bit more real.' In addition, as the writer, star and executive producer of her series, she enjoys the chance to simply focus on performance. 'It is a huge pressure off, acting rather than writing. The writing is the hard pressure to me,' she says ruefully, half way through writing the third series of the sit-com.

Other pleasures include being able to take her Shih-Tzu Peggy to work with her – St Joseph's, the disused seminary where we film, has thirty acres of dog-friendly grounds – and the company of her fellow actors. There is a genuine chemistry between them all. 'It really shows on camera, and it works off camera as well. The cast is a great mix of women who just all gelled. I love them all. It's been lovely to work with them again, making the second series.'

Miranda does take working with tiny infants very seriously. 'The responsibility of working with babies is great. You are holding this priceless newborn, just terrified you are going to drop them.' She adds, 'And they do things like wee in your glove.'

In the final episode of Series One, I wrote a line for Miranda that, when she read it in rehearsal, actually made her punch the air. Told by her mother, Lady Browne, that she must wear white for her forthcoming wedding, Chummy retorts, 'Sorry. No longer entitled.'

She cites this as one of the best things about her role in *Call the Midwife*.

'Getting the man! Now, that was a first.'

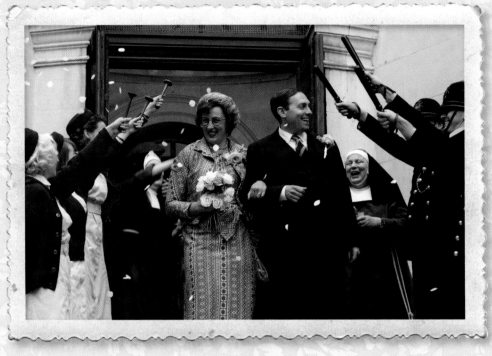

Q&A

What is your favourite outfit?
Last year I made myself a Crimplene skirt suit that I like to wear in church. There's plenty of stretch around the derriere, so it's frightfully comfy, even during quite long sermons.

Where do you go on holiday?
When I was a child in India, I thought there could be no more exotic place on earth than Blackpool, and I still have a soft spot for the seaside. Give me a 99 and a donkey ride, and my heart could burst with joy.

Who is your dream date and where would you go?
Am I allowed to say my husband? And we're both sneakingly fond of a good brass band, so we'd go to Hyde Park bandstand and sit in deckchairs and have tea.

What is your favourite record and film?
It sounds awfully frivolous, but I could listen to Jim Reeves singing 'Chapel In The Moonlight' till the cows come home. And I do love *High Society*, it was the first film Peter and I ever went to together.

What is your most treasured memory?
I slept in the street the night before the Coronation, and got a grandstand view of the procession. Her Majesty waved at me as her carriage went by, I still get a wee bit teary when I think of it.

Your favourite meal?
I do rather relish half a pint of whelks, with bread and butter.

What do you do in your spare time?
Now that I'm married, the ironing.

What's your secret vice?
I sometimes buy a sherbet fountain and guzzle the whole thing without stopping. I suck the sherbet through the liquorice stick and everything. In private, obviously.

And your most shining virtue?
I have unusually warm extremities. My patients like this, and so does my husband.

Where would you like to be in five years' time?
Here. I have never been happier.

PROFILE
+
TRIXIE

In late May 2012, Pippa, Hugh, Philippa and I met for lunch at a restaurant on Piccadilly in London. Our rather special guest was slightly late and we sat craning our necks, with our eyes trained on the door. We wondered if we would recognise her when she arrived. Moments later, there she was – blonde, trim and exquisitely turned out in pink and grey, with a toning hat to top off the ensemble. She looked around, spotted us and gave a confident wave. Any doubt evaporated. It was the real Trixie.

Soon after *Call the Midwife* was broadcast and after Jennifer's death, Pippa had been contacted by Michael Bruce, a British ex-pat living in Switzerland. He revealed that his wife, Antonia, had nursed with Jennifer Worth in Poplar in the late fifties and they believed she had been the inspiration for the character of Trixie. Pippa immediately responded and it was agreed that we would meet when Antonia came to England in the summer.

At first, we were rather nervous. The onscreen Trixie is a little more vampish and colourful than the girl presented in the book, and though Jennifer never objected, it was always possible that Antonia might. But she was, in fact, extremely cordial, clearly understanding the demands of drama, and she said how much she'd liked Helen George's performance.

We were all curious to hear more about Antonia's time 'on the district'. Initially, she said she wasn't sure how much she could remember – her Poplar days were, after all, some fifty years ago. Nevertheless, she had brought with her a leather file containing case notes and photographs from her training days. There were no snaps of Jennifer, but many of Antonia, including one of her looking radiant, fresh-faced – and distinctively blonde

– on a tennis court, posing with some other midwives. It seems extraordinary that they had any energy for sport as their working days were so long and punishing – Antonia once attended three separate deliveries in a single night. In fact, one of her strongest memories is of the sheer grinding hardness of the work. But there is also much that she recalls with joy, including sitting in chapel, listening to the nuns at prayer. Another legacy was a lifetime's friendship with Cynthia, who remained her link to Jennifer after they both married and Antonia had moved abroad.

For actress Helen George, *Call the Midwife* has been all about the formation of close bonds. 'It is a really tight cast and crew who work well together,' she explains. 'I love the scenes when I'm with all the girls – Miranda, Bryony and Jessica – and the delivery scenes are fantastic because there is such a chemistry between us. Then when the nurses relax together, they all eat cake in the Nonnatus House kitchen and Trixie lights up a fag.'

This is perhaps the worst aspect of the job for non-smoker Helen. 'They are herbal cigarettes and they smell awful. No fun at all when you're going for the hundredth take.'

Q&A

What is your favourite outfit?
I think it all begins with the foundations. I couldn't
live without my circle-stitched brassiere and boned
suspender belt.

Where do you go on holiday?
I have a wonderfully indulgent godmother who
lives near Portofino; I try to visit her once a year.

**Who is your dream date and where would
you go?**
I'd find it hard to resist David Niven – older men
are so much more polished. And who could say
no to supper and dancing at the Savoy?

What is your favourite record and film?
I have a Peggy Lee LP that we sometimes play
in the parlour when the nuns have gone to bed.
And I've seen *Love is a Many Splendoured Thing*
five times – there's something so compelling about
a weepie.

What is your most treasured memory?
When I was eight, our cat Blossom had kittens
in my doll's cot. It was the first time I'd witnessed
the miracle of birth – seeds were definitely sown
that day.

Your favourite meal?
Anything eaten in an Italian restaurant, with a red-
checked tablecloth and the company of friends.

What do you do in your spare time?
Mend my stockings and touch up my hair. And
sometimes I sit at the back of the chapel during
Compline and listen to the nuns as they sing their
evening prayers. It touches me in a way I can't
describe.

What's your secret vice?
I read the problem pages in magazines, and give
really rude advice in my head.

And your most shining virtue?
I never show fear.

Where would you like to be in five years' time?
Having fittings for a wedding dress.

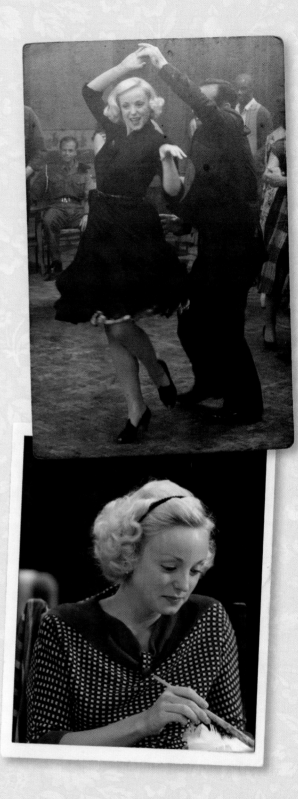

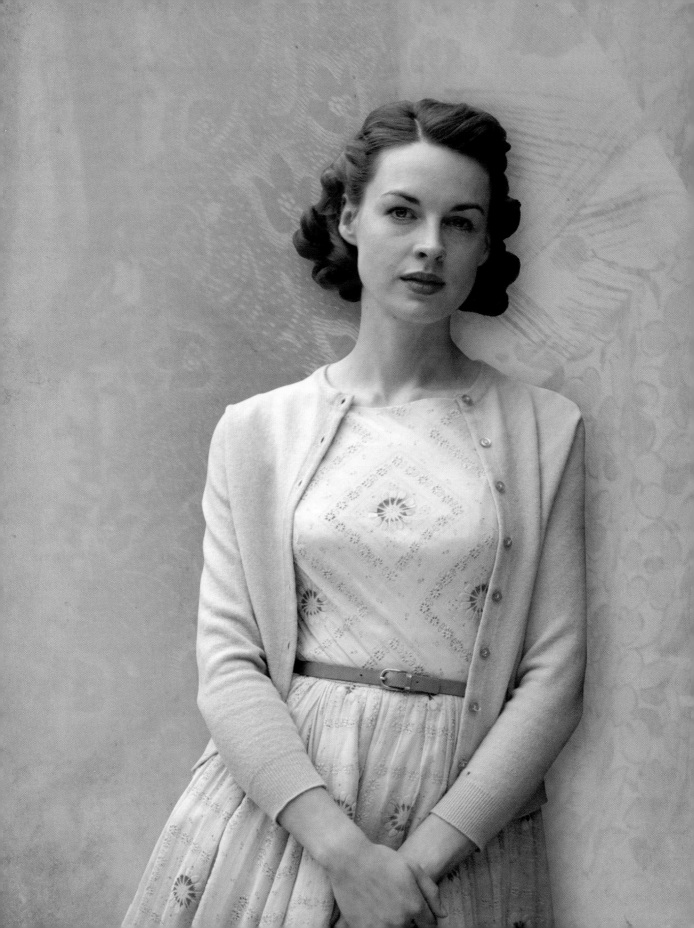

CHAPTER
2
FASHION

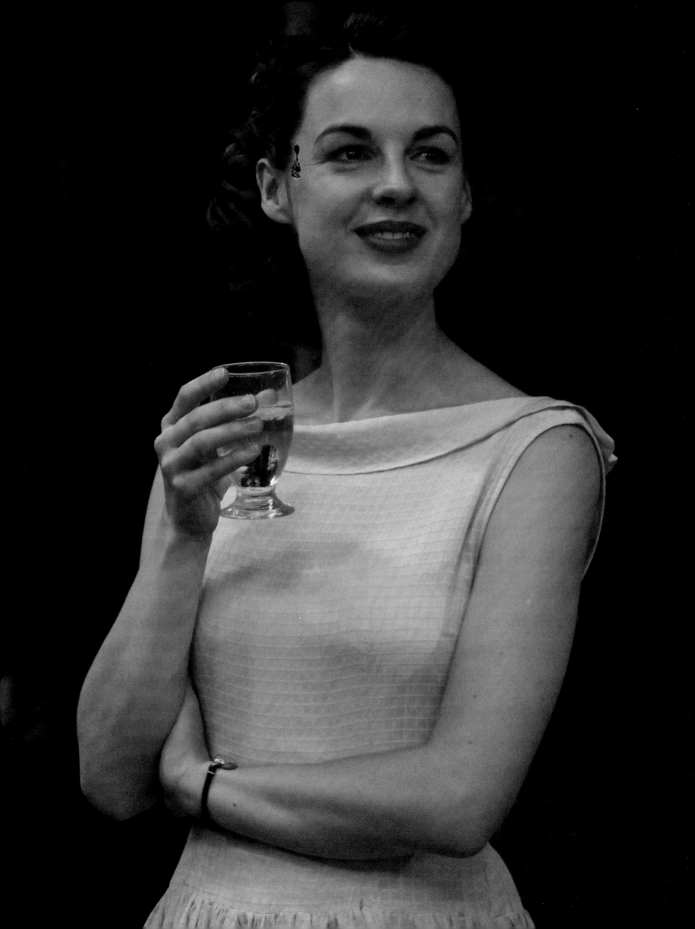

FASHION

Once, when I was on the set of *Cranford*, a very senior actress took exception to the term 'costume drama'. 'Why must people always speak of costume drama?' she asked, in vexed but beautifully modulated tones, 'I wear a costume in everything I'm in!'

She had a point. Costumes are literally woven into the very fabric of every film and television show, be they contemporary or set in the past. As much expertise and care goes into choosing the right jeans and jacket for a cop show as the tippets and gloves of a Gaskell adaptation. But when a drama is set in a different time all aspects of visual design are more immediately apparent and therefore, perhaps, there is more delight to be derived.

I first worked with Amy Roberts on the revival of *Upstairs Downstairs*, for which she received an Emmy nomination for Outstanding Costume Design. When Pippa suggested her for *Call the Midwife*, I knew at once that she'd be absolutely perfect. Amy already had several BAFTA wins for Costume under her belt, including one for the 2007 BBC production of *Oliver Twist* and the previous year's *Elizabeth I: The Virgin Queen*.

One of the most interesting things about *Call the Midwife* is that although it is set long enough ago to qualify as a period drama, the 1950s are within living memory for many of the show's core audience. This throws up challenges for every department, but people remember details of what they and their loved ones were wearing far more vividly than they can recall the finer points of the vehicles in the street or the news on the radio. I knew from the start that we couldn't let the show become a fancy dress parade. And that, to my mind, was why we needed Amy, because she doesn't just do costumes, she does

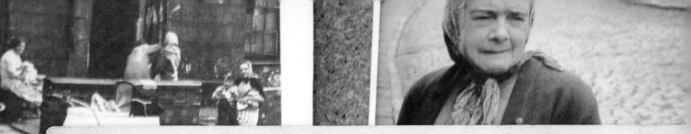

clothes. Detailed, thoughtful, authentic garments that speak of lives lived, and work undertaken. 'These were real people, doing real things, that really happened,' she declares. From the outset, creating complete outfits for every single character from the smallest newborn to the oldest nun, Amy has been passionate in her desire to represent the tough, vibrant people of Poplar. Her determination to do justice to this world comes, in part, from her own family background. Her mother Jo, one of 13 children, grew up in the tough East End district of Custom House and left school when she was just 14 years old.

> *'These were real people, doing real things, that really happened.'*
>
> AMY ROBERTS
> *Costume Designer*

Unfortunately for Amy, her family was one of many at the time that didn't own a camera, so there is no family archive for her to draw upon. However, over the years, she has accrued a wide-ranging personal library of reference material, which includes many photographs, newspapers and magazines from the fifties. Intriguingly, Amy also has a magpie's eye for fashion spreads in the present-day glossies – these often provide clues as to how a character's individual 'look' should be shaped, and give fresh insights into colour and texture. In her files, images torn from *Vogue* rub shoulders with black and white snaps snipped out of *Picture Post*.

Colour is vitally important to Amy. Thanks to the lack of colour images in contemporary journalism and newsreels, it's tempting to think of the fifties as a rather drab decade. This was not necessarily the case, but clothing rationing had only ended in 1949, and less than ten years later many people were in the habit of making 'serviceable' choices in apparel, on the assumption that everything must last. There was still a lot of brown and grey about, and many young men and women were still in military uniform due to the demands of National Service. Amy has developed techniques for making sure the muted tones don't dominate.

'To make a crowd scene more arresting we will throw in an acid-yellow cardigan, or a plum-coloured headscarf to catch the eye. We are making a show and not a documentary.' These small details do much to enliven and enrich the overall visual experience, and can act as a happy antidote to the carefully observed realism of many of the clothes.

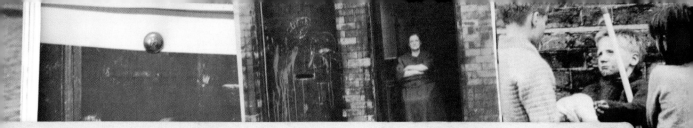

'Nobody looked box-fresh in the fifties,' says Amy. 'If the collar of a bloke's shirt wore out, you would take it off, turn it around and sew it back on. That's what my mum did with my dad's shirts! Or, maybe you had a coat that your mum had made and you either wore it out completely or until it got far too small.'

Amy applied these principles to the Cub pack featured in Series Two. Take a picture of a group of fifties' cub scouts from Amy's extensive collection, for example. A few were proudly wearing full uniform but most were missing some element of it. 'People struggled to save up at the time before buying items like that. One month they would get a cap and the next, a scarf. No one went out and bought everything all in one go,' explains Amy.

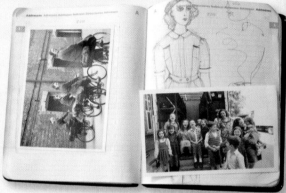

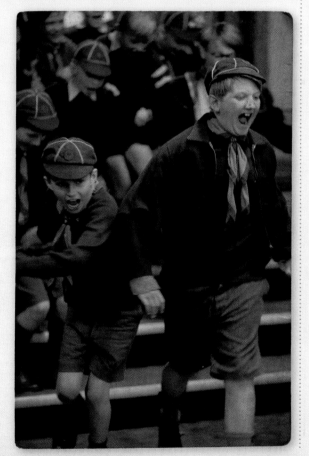

Despite this rigorous authenticity, chances to showcase the more glamorous aspects of fifties' fashion do arise. Popular interest in clothing and style grew throughout the decade, even when many women could only afford to window shop. Jennifer Worth loved the wasp waists and full skirts that swept the world after Christian Dior unveiled the New Look in 1947. In homage to her I created a scene in Series One that shows the young Jenny ironing numerous underskirts in readiness for an outing to a concert at London's Festival Hall. Trixie – svelte in a pencil skirt – pours scorn. 'New Look's old hat, darling!' she opines – and by 1957 it was, but only just.

Although well into her seventies, Coco Chanel had sensed that the tide was turning and steered the market back to slim skirts in 1954. Christian Dior responded with H-, A- and Y-line clothes, with dropped waists, boxy jackets and a generally

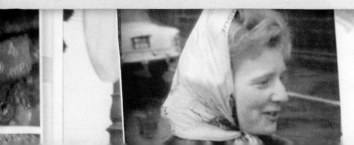

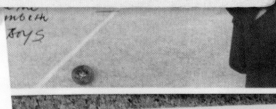

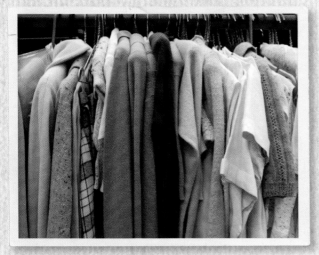

looser fit. One thing led to another, and in 1955
Cristobal Balenciaga presented the tunic dress.
Two years later Hubert de Givenchy introduced
the 'sack', a simple shift that caught on more
slowly, but then endured in popularity for years.

Then, as now, however, personal taste
was more powerful than the dictates of
couturiers, and women used clothes to
express themselves, rather than simply
following the rules. Amy bears this in
mind with every ensemble she creates.
Each principal actor has a wardrobe that
not only reflects the period, but speaks
of the character they play. 'The young
nurses have very distinct personalities,'
explains Amy. 'Their clothes are actually
telling a little bit of their story.'

Jenny Lee's feminine, fawn-like look was
unveiled in her very first scene in the series.
We first see her as a poised but perplexed young
woman picking her way through the heaving
dockside district, struggling with a heavy case.
Jessica Raine was unwell with a bad cough on the

day of filming, which added to her ivory pallor. This, in turn, was complemented by her vintage two-piece suit in beige and white houndstooth and her immaculate stockings and heels.

'Jenny arrives in this extraordinary hubbub of dockworkers. A young middle class girl thrown into this very working class society. That scene triggers her whole look.'

Amy carefully built a palette for Jenny that reflected her restrained femininity, but also suited the actress's porcelain skin. She describes this as, 'Soft and delicate colours, with the occasional olive yellow and chocolate brown thrown in.'

For Cynthia – a quiet but sometimes whimsical young woman, with a hint of hidden depths – the hues tend to be deeper and more mysterious. 'I like her in prune and charcoal, with touches of green,' says Amy. 'She is more quirky than Jenny, perhaps a little bit Prada.'

As for Trixie, the clothes, like the character, are sassy. 'She is gregarious, blonde, feisty and bold enough to wear black. Her outfits have strong, blocked colours that wouldn't look out of place in a jazz club.'

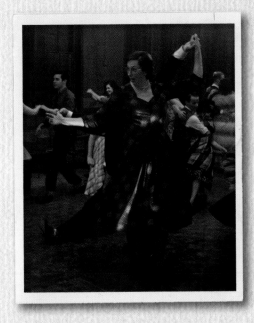

Chummy proved an interesting proposition costume-wise. She has a private income in addition to her nurse's wage, and could purchase a wardrobe that all would envy. But practical Chummy prizes comfort above couture and chooses sensible materials like Crimplene, developed in the fifties as a crease-resistant wash-and-wear fabric. In awe of Amy's expertise, I seldom reference clothing in the scripts, unless it is mentioned in dialogue, but in Series One I chucked in a Crimplene skirt suit without realising that at that time this material was not a by-word for frumpiness but, in fact, quite cutting edge. Amy alerted me to this and, after some discussion, we decided that Crimplene was actually a good social marker for this aristocratic renegade as it was then available only through the smartest establishments.

Chummy has a palette mainly comprised of browns and greys, offset with accents of orange, pink and teal.

> *'The young nurses have very distinct personalities. Their clothes are actually telling a little bit of their story.'*
>
> AMY ROBERTS
> *Costume Designer*

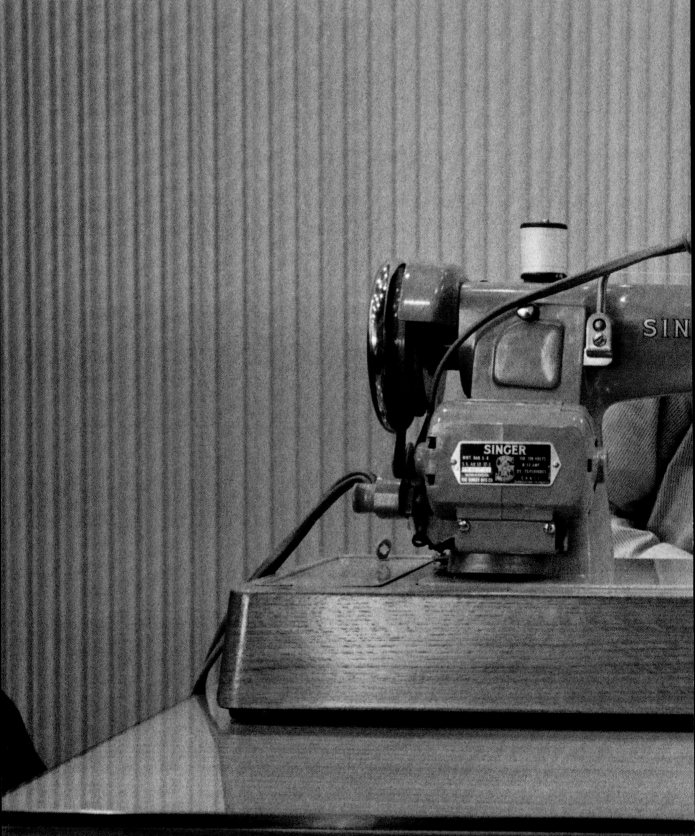

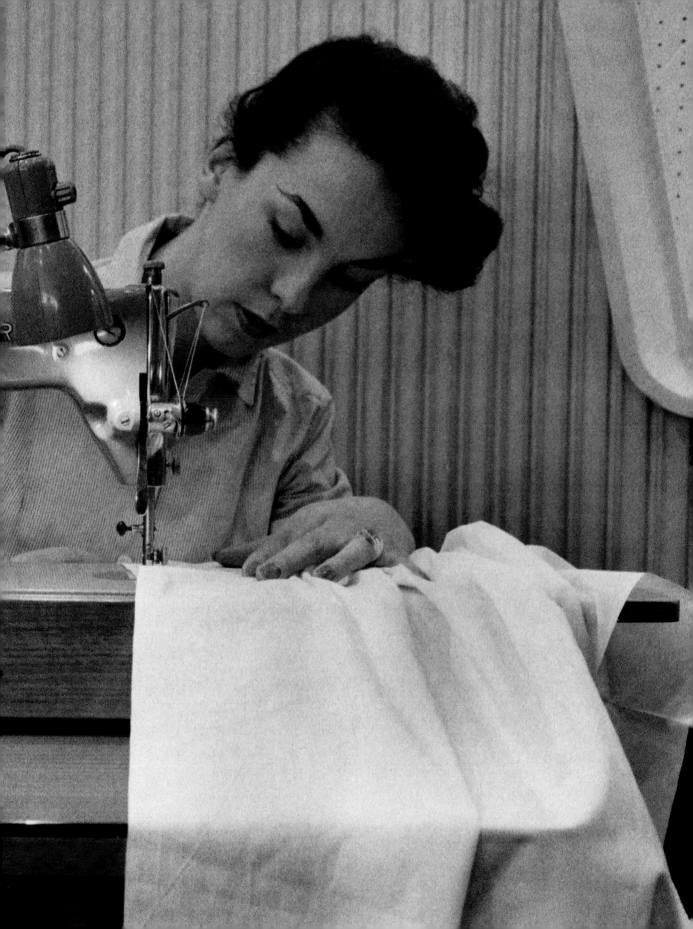

GARROULD'S

Manufacturers of the

National Uniform

for

STATE CERTIFIED MIDWIVES

The Premi... ...d Outfitt...

WE ha...
Uni...
for goo...

YO...
w...
ac...

Hyp...

Where hyperacidity...
patient's distress...
De Witt's Antacid...
tion contains one...
available and h...
mended. For...
acidity, De...
prolonged...
teaspoonf...
a tumbl...
pleasan...
everyw...

ANT... TABLETS for INDIGESTION
flavour. All chemists,
3/2.

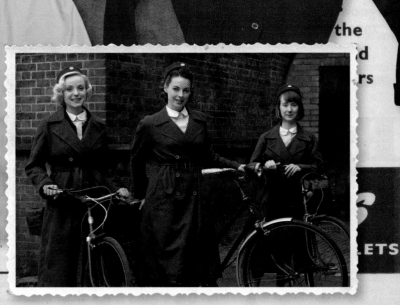

These are colours conservative Chummy might have chosen and they work well with Miranda Hart's lightly tanned complexion and deep hazel eyes. However, a surprise 'gift' of a length of fabric from Sister Monica Joan in Series One offered the chance to extend Chummy's range. For this, Amy chose a glorious turquoise brocade, figured in gold. It had an Indian feel, which was a nice nod to Chummy's childhood in the Raj, but it also seemed to hint that Chummy was setting sail for pastures new and that her life was opening out.

In the story, she makes herself a dress from the cloth to wear for her momentous meeting with PC Noakes' parents. She then ruins it by becoming involved in the surprise delivery of a litter of piglets. Amy made two dresses in order to accommodate this storyline. One had to be pristine, the other smothered in Nutella – to represent lashings of pig manure.

It is not unusual for costumes to be created in duplicate, especially with frequently worn items such as uniforms. In *Call the Midwife* the nurses' outfits and the nuns' habits work exceptionally hard, and if a piece of clothing is torn or stained it needs to be replaced – often at a moment's notice – with an identical item.

The nurses' working clothes and the nuns' habits were all created from scratch by Amy after she carefully balanced painstaking research with the needs of the television medium. The uniforms worn by the real-life midwives were predominantly grey, but this would have looked very drab on screen. Amy compromised, keeping the belted, grey gabardines and choosing a soft blue for the dresses, with a crisp white Peter Pan collar. There was debate about the headgear: as young midwives, Jennifer Worth and her colleagues sported grey felt boaters, but these would do no one any favours. Eventually the team settled on a brimless hat in cherry red with cardigan to match, the latter a nod to the chilly domestic conditions in which nurses often worked.

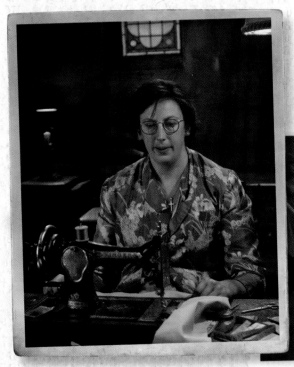

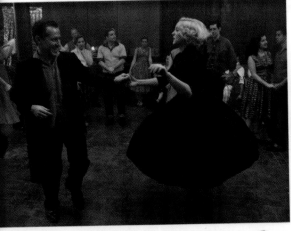

The hosiery proved interesting – it transpired that the sheer black stockings of popular memory were either a later arrival or the product of the collective male imagination. Stout tan nylons were the order of the day in Poplar in the fifties, worn with saddle-brown lace-up shoes.

> *'The religious habit wasn't at all suitable for the work we had to do as midwives. What we needed was a pair of slacks.'*
>
> SISTER CHRISTINE HOVERD
> *The Community of St John the Divine*

Research for the nuns' habits involved a trip to Birmingham. Here, Amy and director Philippa Lowthorpe met with the Sisters of the Order of St John the Divine – the inspiration for the Order of St Raymond Nonnatus in the series. Though the Sisters no longer wear the habit, they had an entire, carefully preserved ensemble tucked away. This comprised the basic dress or tunic, the scapula, which is a tabard-like outer garment, and the wimple and veil. Amy was able to turn the garments inside out and collate information about how they were structured and made. Then Philippa modelled the wimple and veil, so that all details about fastenings and so forth could be carefully recorded.

The original habit was a surprisingly vibrant saxe blue. Unusually, the warmth and depth of the shade were deemed too strong to work on screen, so Amy had to tone it down. She selected

instead a more subdued, monastic blue, which still worked well with the crisp, short veils. The habits clear the ground by several inches, but there was still some consternation as to how the nuns would ride their bikes. Sister Teresa French, who is now 93, provided the answer, 'We used to tuck our scapulas in our belts!' The eagle-eyed can spot Pam Ferris doing exactly this, every time Sister Evangelina mounts her bike.

Sister Christine and Sister Margaret-Angela, of the Community of St John the Divine, both worked in Poplar at much the same time as Jennifer Worth. Along with Sister Teresa, they feature in many archive photographs of the Order in the early 1960s, wearing the habit and veil. They are philosophical about the nuns' move away from traditional garb. Sister Christine explains, 'The religious habit was based on the ordinary dress of the time, which was basically medieval! Looking back, it wasn't at all suitable for a lot of the work we had to do as midwives. What you needed was a pair of slacks.'

Although the Sisters no longer practise as midwives, they still opt for practical clothing in the present day. They sport no-nonsense blouses, skirts and trousers in styles of their own choosing, and make many of their clothes themselves. This is partly a nod to their vow of poverty, but is a sensible economy that would be recognisable to many a woman in the fifties.

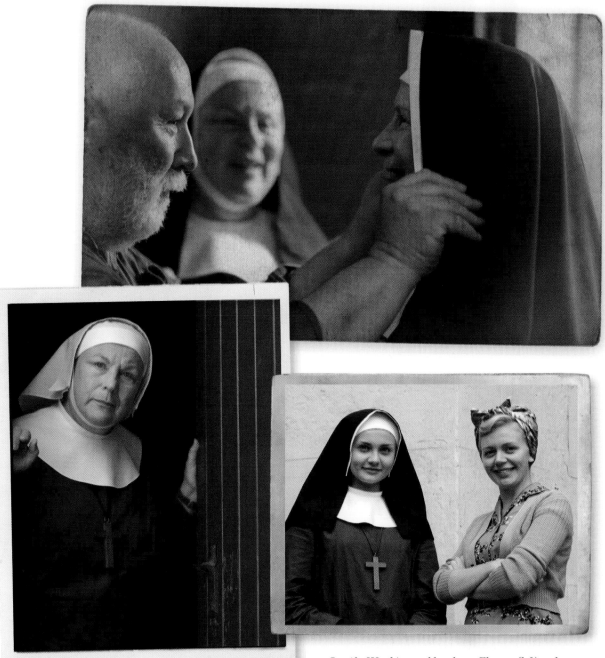

Jennifer Worth's granddaughters, Eleanor (left) and Lydia (right), dressed as extras for Chummy's wedding.

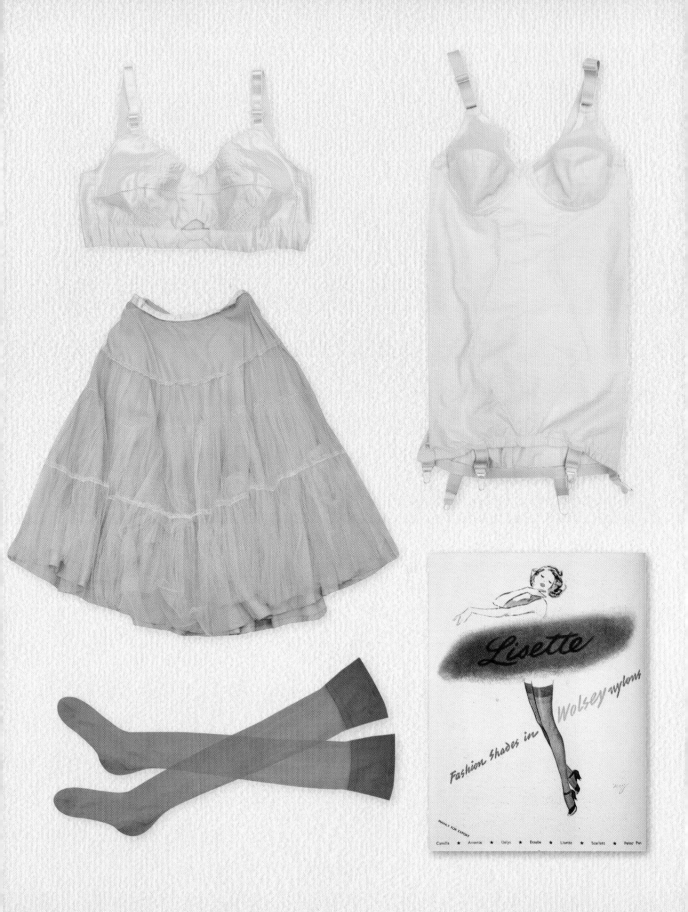

'LAUGHTER, LOVE AND LINGERIE'

Miranda Hart

CHUMMY

Home dressmaking was commonplace in the years before and after the War, as much out of necessity as for the fun of it. An electric Singer sewing machine was a big investment, but many families had pedal-powered workhorses handed down by the previous generation. Material and trimmings were relatively inexpensive and shops carried a wide range of paper patterns. These were often at the vanguard of fashion.

One particular pattern, for the Walk-Away Dress, was so popular that it is even credited with the post-war recovery of American company Butterick's. The advertising for the pattern promised, 'Start it after breakfast – walk away in it for luncheon!' The simple, wrap-around design became ubiquitous in wardrobes throughout Britain and the States.

There were patterns for everything, including gloves, petticoats and even bras. Industrious, hard-up women sometimes had access to parachute silk left over from the War, which they could turn into glamorous undergarments. They might eventually take the scissors to a satin wedding gown for the same discreet purpose (if they hadn't already dyed it and remade it as a dance dress). Underwear is a key part of the *Call the Midwife* costume experience, just as it was vital to real women at the time.

'The girls in the show love it,' says Amy. 'It is like putting on a fifties' skin. They say it makes them feel absolutely right for the part.'

Some of the underwear dates back sixty years, though good-quality replica items are increasingly available through specialist outlets. 'You have got to get the bosoms in the right place,' Amy adds. 'In the fifties, they were high up and cone shaped, due to the invention of the bullet bra.'

> *Underwear is a key part of the* Call the Midwife *costume experience, just as it was vital to real women at the time.*

This sought-after silhouette was largely popularised by the 'Sweater Girl' pin-ups of the day, most notably Lana Turner and Jane Russell. Only after Lycra appeared in 1959 did smooth bras become popular, although Amy was able to source a very plain, soft cotton brassiere for Sister Bernadette that would never be seen – or even hinted at – beneath the habit. Actress Laura Main became surprisingly attached to this. 'I love my plain bra and my big pants. It says so much to me about Bernadette, how her whole life was about work and service, and not at all to do with vanity or even being especially feminine.' Between Series One and Two the bra went missing, to Laura's dismay, and when it was eventually returned to her she felt she was greeting a much-loved friend.

The nuns wore thick black woollen or cotton hose held up with elastic garters, which constricted circulation and could cause varicose veins. Most ordinary women chose stockings and suspenders. The suspenders were generally attached to a heavy elasticated girdle or corselette. These foundations were popularly known as a 'roll-on' as they were designed to be rolled up and over the abdomen by the wearer. It was often a rather tight squeeze! While constricting undergarments like these were abandoned during the more free-and-easy seventies and eighties, since the rise of modern elastane fabrics, 'shapewear' is once again in vogue.

'We are going back to this style now, with underwear that smoothes everything out,' observes Amy. 'It also gives you a mono bottom; one curve like Marilyn Monroe rather than two distinct cheeks.'

All dramas, period or otherwise, must operate within a budget and, despite its ambitious scale and large cast, *Call the Midwife* is no exception. The costume department garners its resources carefully. Some clothes are individually commissioned from specialist tailors, while others are run up on the premises by the team.

Costume supervisor Peter Halston reveals, 'We make the simple items – anything without a collar, including hospital gowns, negligées and so forth. Also some of these costumes are sixty years old. They fall apart, and we patch them up.'

In addition to chance finds in thrift shops and at antique clothing markets, many vintage pieces are to be found for hire on the rails of London's theatrical costumiers such as Cosprop or Angels. Amy and Assistant Costume Designer Emma Moore spend many hours rifling through row upon row of garments, in search of precisely the right items. Original fifties' hats, coats, dresses, trousers, skirts, waistcoats, shirts and shoes can be found in these costumiers in

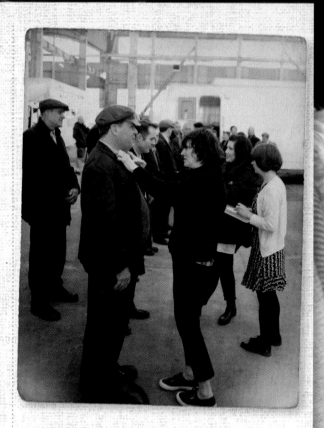

Amy and Assistant Costume Designer Emma Moore spend many hours rifling through row upon row of garments, in search of precisely the right items.

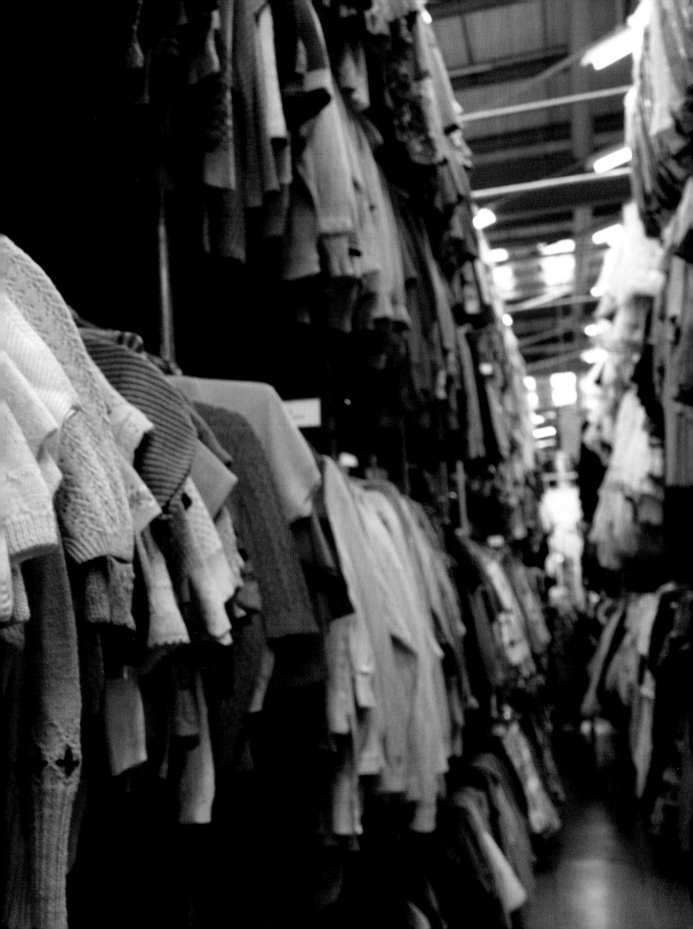

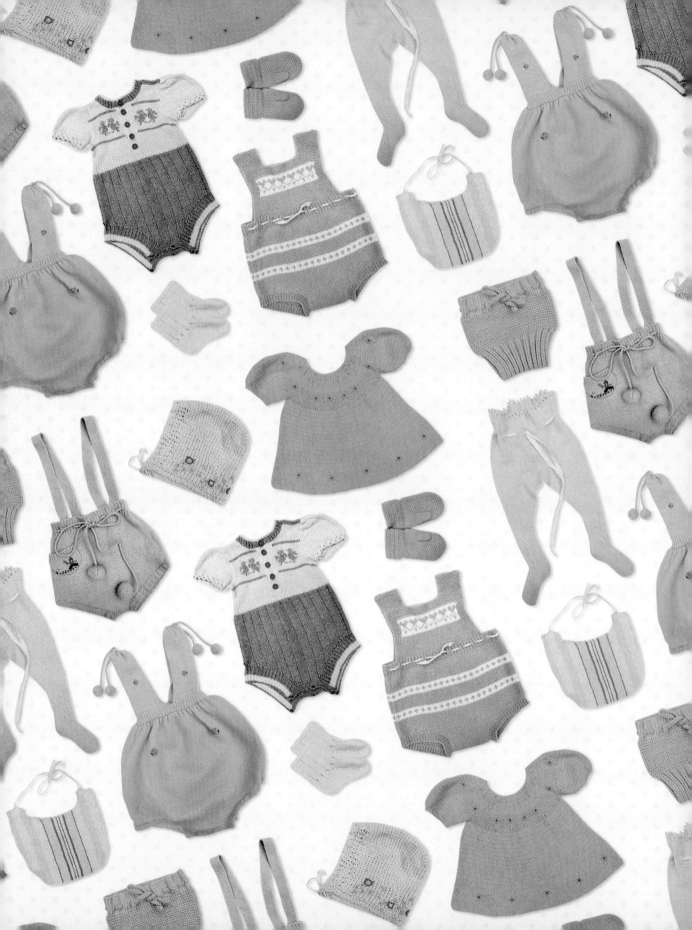

abundance – each neatly labelled with details of its previous appearances on the screen. Sometimes a long-gone actor's name or monogram may even be stitched on the lining of a jacket. Stephen McGann, who plays Dr Turner, finds Angels a magical place.

'There is such a sense of history about those clothes. Not just fashion history, but the history of the entertainment industry itself. The clothes are handed down from one generation of performers to the next – there's that sense of literally walking in the shoes of other actors, and it's very special.'

The costumes on the show must be carefully maintained. In addition to running repairs, the laundry is never ending. Stockings are mended as required and washed every day. One of my favourite sights on the *Call the Midwife* set is the rack of damp nylons blowing lightly in the breeze outside the wardrobe trailer.

Other costumes are laundered once a week, on site, and there are two irons to hand in case one of them malfunctions. In the main, the routine runs like clockwork, but once in a while there are moments of panic. The most memorable of these moments was when Miranda's nurses' uniform needed a quick freshen up between scenes.

'It came out lovely and clean,' said Peter Halston, who had popped it in the washing machine. 'Then, as I shook it out, a bit of plastic fell on to the floor. I went cold.'

The 'bit of plastic' was a lens from Chummy's glasses, which had been slipped into a pocket for safekeeping. They were an original fifties pair – very possibly the last frames of the kind still in existence. A major continuity disaster loomed.

It was all hands on deck at *Call the Midwife*. While an assistant rang every optical outlet in the southeast, hoping to find a replacement pair of glasses, the shooting schedule was realigned to buy time. After a frantic search, Peter located the other lens and the metal frame inside the body of the washer, but large sections of its fractured Bakelite coating were missing, and the specs remained unwearable.

'Eventually we lifted up the machine and performed a Caesarean section on the waste pipe to retrieve the last of the Bakelite splinters. Then we stuck the glasses back together. The glue was still wet when Miranda went back in front of the camera.'

Peter still winces at the memory, but adds, 'There's no point in screaming and shouting. What's great about this show is that everybody holds out a hand to get you back on the lifeboat.'

Call the Midwife has a voracious appetite for vintage-style baby knits, once the prop and mainstay of every infant's wardrobe.

Call the Midwife is sustained by many other pairs of unseen hands. For example, the show has a voracious appetite for vintage-style baby knits, once the prop and mainstay of every infant's wardrobe. My Grandma – a peerless knitter who could conjure up complex Aran designs without referring to a pattern – made it her business to kit out every newborn in the family with a full layette in 3-ply wool. 'I like to see a baby in handknits,' she said very firmly, when informed that handknits had had their day. 'They make them look loved.'

Unsurprisingly, there are only a few examples of vintage knitted children's clothes available today. Even the most cherished cardigans were subject to moth attack, or passed on when outgrown, then discarded several babies down the line. In the 1980s I remember seeing a baby's pram coat with its hem stitched up, hung on a back door, doing duty as a peg bag.

Babies also rock a vintage look with their nether garments — terry towelling nappies are the order of the day.

Once knitted garments are acquired by Amy and her team, they are recycled across episodes and among the tiny actors. An armoury of matelot hats, matinée jackets and balaclava helmets is steadily building in size. Amy commissions many pieces from Sandra Sell, who runs a wool shop in Clacton-on-Sea in Essex. Sandra, in turn, has willing helpers who can turn their hand to nostalgia knitting.

'Those knitters own a little bit of this show, and they are very proud to be involved with it, which is lovely,' says Peter.

The *Call the Midwife* babies also rock a vintage look with their nether garments – terry towelling nappies are the order of the day. Amy and her team pin the nappies on over ordinary disposables. The resulting bulkiness is entirely appropriate for the period because, as Amy explains, those mums who could afford to were already lining the towelling squares with Paddi Pads, a forerunner of the disposable nappy. Made of cellulose and cotton wool, these helped save on laundry and went some way towards preventing nappy rash. The clip-on plastic pants designed to hold the pads in place were less popular, because they were inclined to leak and cause skin irritation.

But plastic had commenced its march and, with its chemically engineered stablemate nylon, it was poised to revolutionise fashion. Accessories such as bags, shoes and gloves – considered essential for even the youngest ladies in the fifties – were traditionally made from leather. Plastic began to edge leather off the shelves and bring prices down in the process.

Meanwhile, nylon clothes were simple to wash, quick to dry and required no ironing. Those advantages outweighed nylon's slithering, uncomfortable feel and tendency to spark minute electric charges. As nylon became affordable, it was embraced by old and young alike.

So, gradually, everything changed. Because it always does. Fashion, by very definition, shifts its shape with the passage of time.

Running my hands along the racks of clothes in the *Call the Midwife* wardrobe, I am touched by the sense of the people who once wore them or whose lives our series conjures up. A flowered blouse, a peach silk slip, a mended waistcoat. A pair of toddler's dungarees, an apron, a bridal gown. These are clothes that were chosen, worn with pleasure or a sense of compromise. The armour in which their owners faced the day.

And the conclusion is inescapable: everybody's life is a costume drama, really.

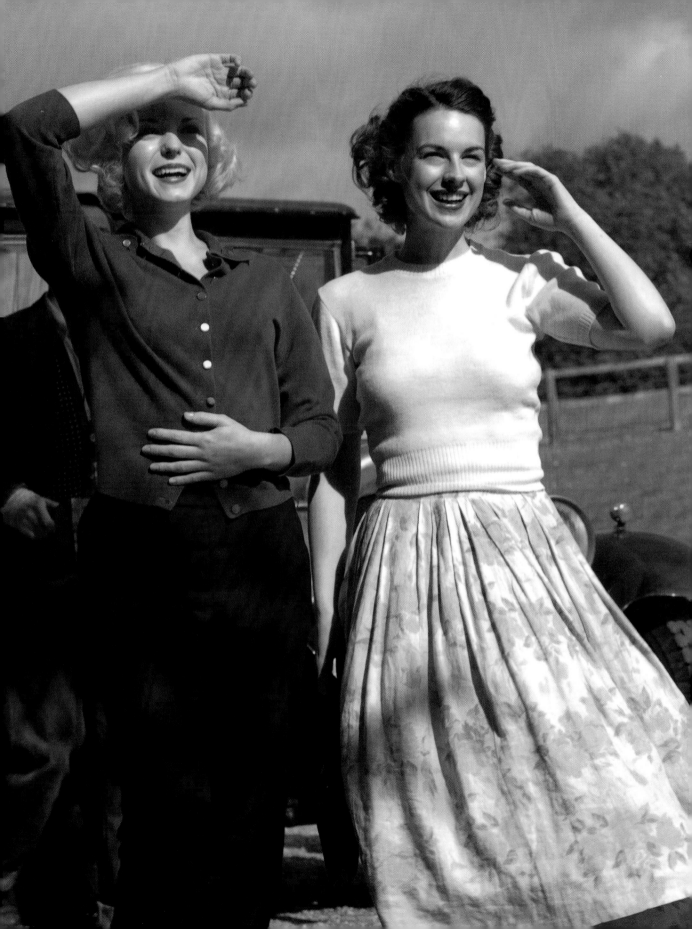

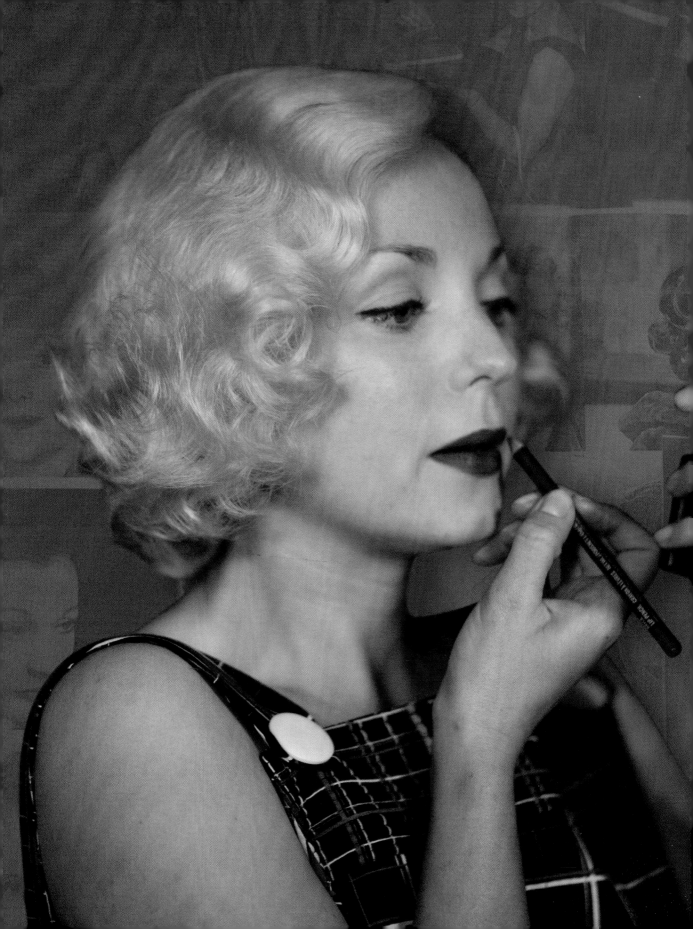

CHAPTER
3

Beauty

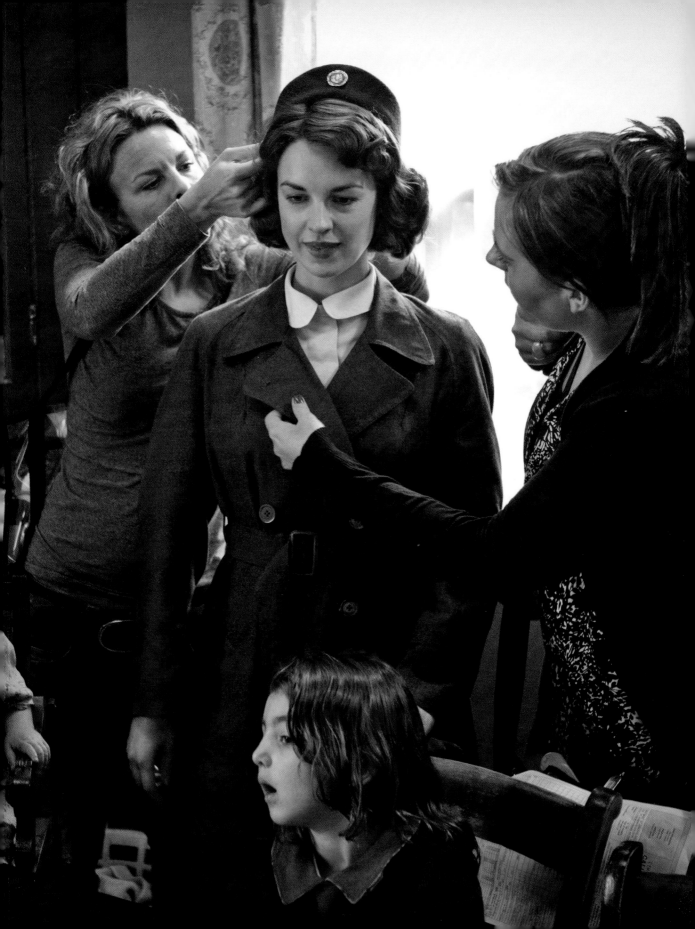

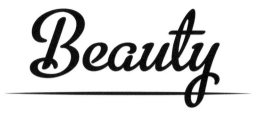

Beauty

'I HAVE THIS FANTASY ABOUT PAINTING MY NAILS.
CHERRY-RED TALONS, GLEAMING IN THE LIGHT.
ONE DAY I WON'T BE ABLE TO RESIST IT ANY MORE.'

Trixie

I sometimes think a quick flick through a vintage women's magazine can tell you more about female experience than a shelf full of history books. The pages on beauty – be they advertising features, or how-to columns – are often the most evocative. The way we are supposed to paint our lips or shape our brows seems to shift and change not just from decade to decade, but from year to year.

Yet we all cling to cosmetics we love, whether they fit the current ideal or not. A mere lipstick colour can become a talisman. Rimmel's Gay Geranium, launched in 1935, was a bestseller for seventy years – my own aunt favoured it, as did her mother before her. A bright orangey red, it is meant to be outmoded, but thousands of women deem it indispensable. Its recent abrupt withdrawal from the market caused uproar. Rimmel bowed to pressure and restored it to the shelves.

In short, hair and make-up matter; they say much about the times we live in, but even more about the way we see ourselves. And I believe that *Call the Midwife* isn't solely about birth; it is also about what it means, and meant, to be a woman. Getting the hair and make-up right was, to my mind, an essential part of the mission of the show.

I was thrilled when producer Hugh Warren and principal director Philippa Lowthorpe persuaded Christine Walmesley-Cotham to join the team. Her past credits include major historical dramas such as *Vanity Fair* and *Miss Austen Regrets*, so we knew we were in safe hands.

Christine constantly looks to archive material for her inspiration. Scattered around the make-up trailer are a 1958 copy of *Vogue*, along with fifties editions of *Picturegoer* and *Woman's Journal*.

'A huge part of achieving a look is getting the hair right. In addition to waistlines, the volume and lustre of our hair is perhaps where the greatest changes have been, style-wise, in the past 60 years.'

She says that hair is her biggest daily challenge. The nuns are quickly despatched – one starched wimple pinned in place, and they're ready to go. But what of Jenny, Chummy, Trixie and Cynthia? Guest characters such as Spanish Conchita Warren and Mary, the teenage prostitute? There are also dozens of extras in each episode, and these too must be styled in the manner of the day.

'A huge part of achieving the look is getting the hair right. In addition to waist lines, the volume and lustre of our hair is perhaps where the greatest changes have been, style-wise, in the past 60 years.'

Christine Walmesley-Cotham
Hair and Make-up Designer

Christine tries, as far as possible, to work with each actress's natural hair. It is not always easy as today's styles tend towards long and straight, while in the fifties, hairdos were usually short and curls were in vogue. As ever, celebrities led the way. Queen Elizabeth II and Elizabeth Taylor inspired the masses with their neat bouncy bubble cuts, though few sought to copy Lucille Ball's poodle wave.

In the first series of *Call the Midwife*, Jessica Raine's soft brown hair was cut and permed for the role of Jenny Lee. In order to look professional under a nurse's cap, it was then held back from her face with kirby grips. For the second series, the decision was taken not to replicate this style. 'This time Jenny's hair was a bit longer, and also slightly straighter, to imply the passing of time,' explained Christine.

Perhaps we will see it cut shorter in due course – as the fifties tipped towards the sixties, Audrey Hepburn popularised a short, gamine style with an urchin fringe. But the silver screen has already inspired the look of one of our leads.

When Helen George auditioned for the role of Trixie, there were three things about her that struck me as quite perfect for the part. The first was her cut-glass accent, the second her comic timing and the third her peroxide blonde coiffure. I was afraid that it might not be possible to keep it, but Christine thought the look just right. Helen's bleached locks exactly match the shade popularised by fifties' pin-ups, such as Jayne Mansfield and Diana Dors.

'Helen's own colour is entirely acceptable, because her character is extrovert enough to have copied a film star.'

Nevertheless, Christine keeps an eagle eye out for anything that screams '2012'. Sixty years ago, highlighting was unknown. If an extra arrives with fashionable streaks, Christine often applies a temporary colour, robust enough to give the hair a solid hue. It won't ruin an expensive salon job, however, and after filming ends it washes out within the week.

In the 21st century, red rinses and highlights are universally popular. These too have to be erased for the cameras. 'So many modern hair colours are new,' comments Christine. 'All those

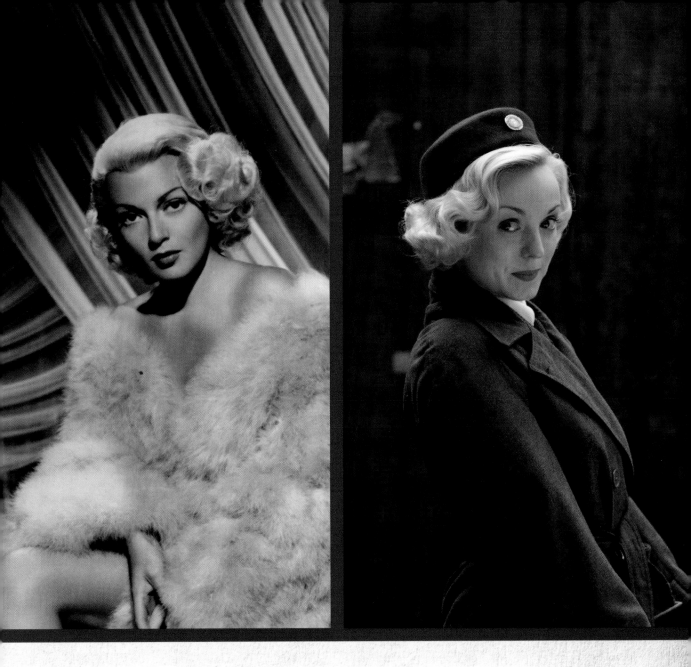

The Film Star Look

'Helen's own colour is entirely acceptable,
because her character is extrovert enough
to have copied a film star.'

reds we see on the high street are modern reds. In the fifties, henna would have been around, but not in any great quantity.'

If matters have gone beyond chemical disguise, Christine turns to her extensive wig collection. Wigs are treasured within the film and television industry, often made over, and never discarded lightly. Leading actresses may ask if a wig worn on a previous job can be tracked down and adapted for a different part. Most hair designers are glad to do this – and the reason is simple.

'To have a full wig made from scratch costs in the region of £1,500,' explains Christine. 'They are handmade and it is a labour-intensive job. Each strand of hair is knotted on to a lacy skull cap, which will blend into the skin when it is put on. The makers will use a blend of four different colours, because we all have at least that many shades in our hair.'

Wigs like these are the exception, not the rule. On a busy show like *Call the Midwife*, the designers have to be pragmatic. The cheaper option is a single-colour, machine-made wig. However, if an extra is to be seen in close-up, it can be preferable to use a 'three-quarter' hairpiece. This disguises the back of the actor's hair, while the natural fringe is carefully styled to match – and hide the join.

One surprising issue, be it with coloured or natural hair, or a wig, is shine. The glossy, light-reflecting sheen we favour in the present day is entirely wrong for 1958. 'We are all so clean, shiny and sparkling now. I'm not saying that people were dirty in the fifties, but they didn't have the products we use today,' says Christine.

Hair was routinely washed with soap until the 1930s, when the first commercial shampoos became available. One of the earliest and most enduring brands was Silvikrin, whose adverts urged women to 'Wash new pep into tired hair'. The hair was probably looking tired because it was frequently home-permed and washed, but only once a week or less. When wet, it was styled with lotions ranging from Amami Wave Set to plain old sugar and water, mixed to a low-cost paste in the kitchen. As Christine observes, 'Those women wouldn't have had a great deal of money to spend on themselves, but they still wanted to look nice.'

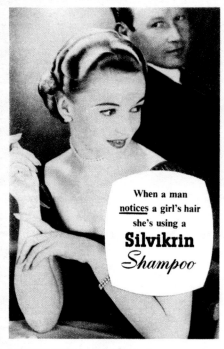

When a man **notices** a girl's hair she's using a **Silvikrin** *Shampoo*

EVERY TIME you use a Silvikrin shampoo you're giving yourself the surest promise of glowing, silky hair—hair that captivates by its sheer loveliness! You see, every Silvikrin shampoo, whether powder, liquid or cream, is enriched with *Pure Silvikrin*, and brings new health and beauty into every single strand of your hair. For hair that men will notice, use a Silvikrin shampoo—and make *certain* of perfect hair health!

C.S.1

• **POWDER** 4½d • **LIQUID** 6d and 1/5d • **CREAM** 1/5d and 2/3d •

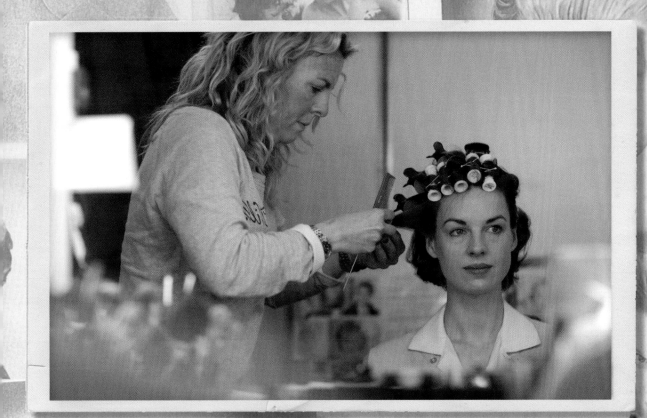

The hair was then wrapped around metal or plastic rollers, fixed with pins and swathed in a scarf or net for several hours. Once the hair was dry, results were guaranteed to last. An advert for Amami promised, 'The loveliest waves that stay set for days. Never an off-looking moment!'

The brutal regime of fixative and rollers may well have led in due course to the emergency purchase of a tube of Vitapointe, a cream massaged into the hair to restore softness. Conditioner for damaged tresses was unknown (though those with dandruff might seek succour in Medicated Vosene), and if all else failed it was back to the kitchen – for an egg. Fresh raw egg, rubbed in well, provided a primitive protein treatment, though care had to be taken in the rinsing out. If the water was too hot, the end result was not silken hair, but a scalp full of omelette.

Flower brand

BEST QUALITY
名花牌发夹 HAIR GRIPS

For 'How to Do', see next page.
TOO GLAM !

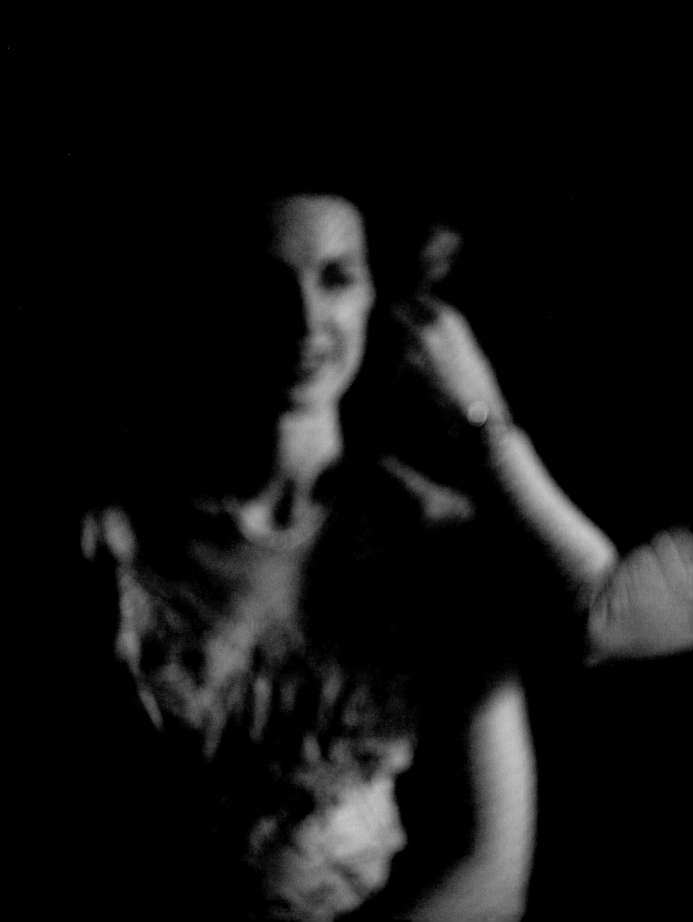

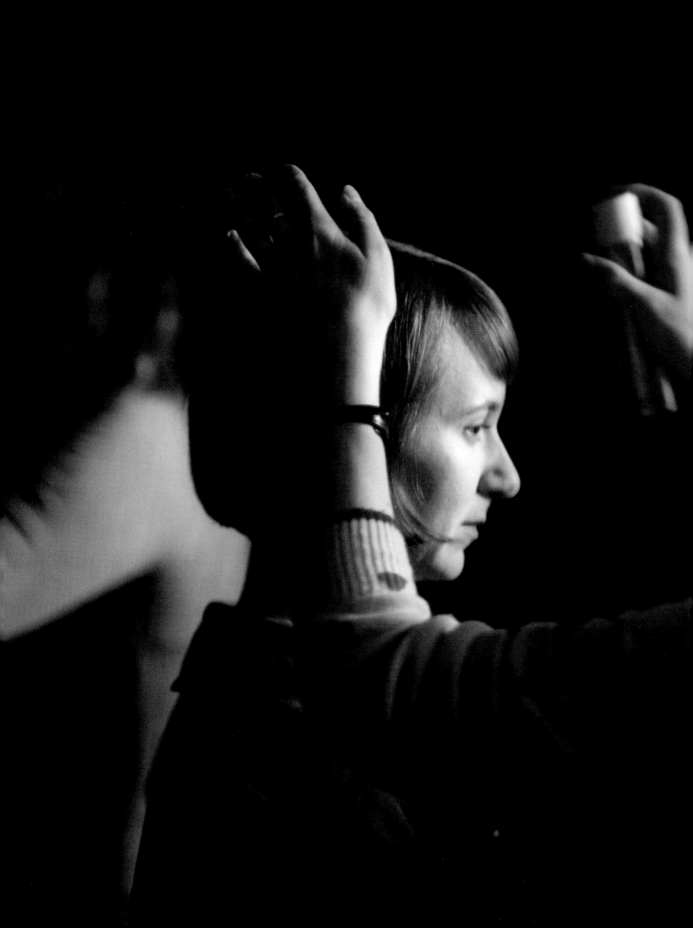

Drying could also prove quite problematic. The first hairdryer had been invented in 1890 – a vast and stationary device that sucked rather than blew the water from the hair of the woman sitting underneath it. The inaugural hand-held models were made from metal, woefully feeble and impossibly cumbersome to use. Only in the 1960s, when the plastics revolution made its way into the home, did lightweight dryers come onto the market. In the meantime, people improvised.

In the twenties and thirties, drying hair with the air outlet or 'exhaust pipe' of a vacuum cleaner was an established practice. And in the mid-fifties my mother, then a young woman, called on a friend who had just been dumped by her fiancé. Entering the kitchen, she was appalled to see her kneeling on the floor with her head inside the oven. My mother, fearing suicide, leaped into action and dragged her out, only to have her friend protest – with her hair full of pincurls – 'I'm drying me hair!'

Men did not generally go to such lengths with their personal grooming, and this is reflected in the way we style the chaps in *Call the Midwife*. They are clean-shaven, in the main, and hair is kept short, especially at the back. Handyman Fred keeps his clipped almost to stubble all over – a legacy of his military roots, perhaps. Meanwhile, Jimmy, Jenny's young beau, is styled with a bit more length on top and a barely detectable dab of Brylcreem.

Brylcreem – a blend of water, mineral oil and beeswax – had been around for some years, but grew in popularity in the fifties. Although its original promise was to bring 'new life to dry hair', over the decade it became a styling aid. Larger and larger amounts were used, despite an early advert claiming, 'A little dab'll do ya'. A new trend evolved, at first confined to Teddy Boys, in which the hair was swept up at the back, brushed over the head, and coaxed into a flicked and rolled quiff. This was commonly known as a DA, and there was some debate as to whether this meant 'district attorney' or 'duck's a*se'.

Elaborate male hairstyles did gain some ground. Sculpted waves became generally desirable, to the point where a children's product,

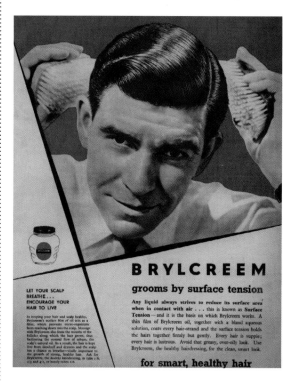

LET YOUR SCALP BREATHE . . . ENCOURAGE YOUR HAIR TO LIVE

In keeping your hair and scalp healthy, Brylcreem's surface film of oil acts as a filter, which prevents micro-organisms from reaching down into the scalp. Massage with Brylcreem also frees the mouths of the follicles along which the hair grows, thus facilitating the normal flow of sebum, the scalp's natural oil. As a result, the hair is kept free from dandruff and dryness and the scalp has a chance to breathe—vitally important to the growth of strong, healthy hair. Ask for Brylcreem, the healthy hairdressing, in tube 2/6, 4/9 and 9/6, or handy tubes 1/0.

BRYLCREEM

grooms by surface tension

Any liquid always strives to reduce its surface area when in contact with air . . . this is known as Surface Tension—and it is the basis on which Brylcreem works. A thin film of Brylcreem oil, together with a bland aqueous solution, coats every hair-strand and the surface tension holds the hairs together firmly but gently. Every hair is supple; every hair is lustrous. Avoid that greasy, over-oily look. Use Brylcreem, the healthy hairdressing, for the clean, smart look.

for smart, healthy hair

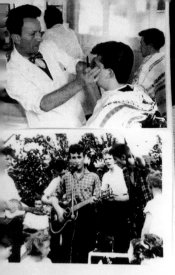

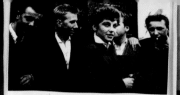

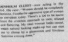

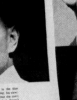

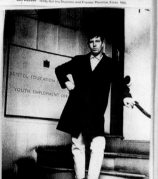

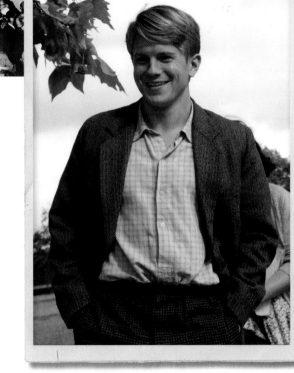

Toddilox, was launched. At a costly two shillings and tuppence h'apenny per jar, it needed to convince potential customers. 'It's safe to say,' trumpeted the advert, 'that Toddilox DOES curl baby's hair, no matter how straight it is now!'

We might feature the odd Toddiloxed infant, but the Teddy Boys and their ilk are shadowy figures in *Call the Midwife*, glimpsed only in the background, never taking centre stage. Our focus is on men who have settled down and are fathering children, or are linked to the women of Nonnatus House.

Stephen McGann, who plays Dr Turner, sports a neat and conservative short back and sides for his role. On glimpsing himself in the mirror for the first time, he was surprised to find he felt quite moved. 'It was like looking at my father, and as if my father was looking back at me.'

George Rainsford, who played Jimmy in Series One.

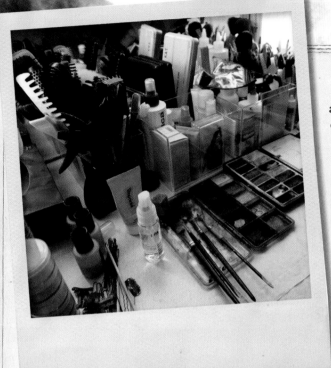

Once the hair is in place, it is time for make-up. For Christine and her fellow artists the work for *Call the Midwife* is quite straightforward.

Sisters Julienne, Monica Joan, Bernadette and Evangelina don't appear to use cosmetics but as Christine confides, 'There's just enough to cover any blemishes.' There's an almost imperceptible amount of colour on their cheeks and a touch of salve to smooth their lips.

Most of the time, our midwives are almost equally bare faced. Lipstick was forbidden when in nursing uniform, but even discreet foundation and mascara were unlikely to be worn. As Christine points out, 'They would have been too busy to apply make-up when they were working.' Only when they head for the pictures or a dance do our heroines plump for colour – unless, like Cynthia, they lack the confidence.

When the girls go out in mufti, greens, blues and turquoises are the colours of choice for eyes, with orangey reds to emphasise the lips. Chummy, played by Miranda Hart, has been known to splash out in the lip department, sporting a slick of bright red on her wedding day. History failed to record whether it was Gay Geranium.

Interestingly, in the fifties, lipstick played more than one role in the beauty routine. Blusher is now a stock item in a woman's handbag, but it's a very new arrival, according to Christine. 'Women would have put a little bit of lipstick on their cheeks. My mother used to make her own rouge with old lipsticks that she put into a saucepan, melted down and then kept in a screw-topped jar to rub on to her face,' she recalls.

Christine uses modern products on the *Call the Midwife* cast. Gone are the days of solid-block mascara, which had to be mixed with the user's spit, and worked to a paste with a miniature brush. Gone, too, are the blocks of greasy panstick and compacts of matte chalky powder. The latest foundations and concealers have far more to offer in terms of finish. With the advent of high definition technology, which can cruelly highlight any flaw or imperfection, this is of paramount importance. A make-up artist's work is at its best when it's invisible.

Achieving naturalism is important in another branch of Christine's work. She and her team are responsible for all the medical effects and prostheses on the show. As the staff at Nonnatus House is not just midwives but also district nurses, the challenges are varied – everything from wounds to pregnant bellies and the occasional corpse. In Series One,

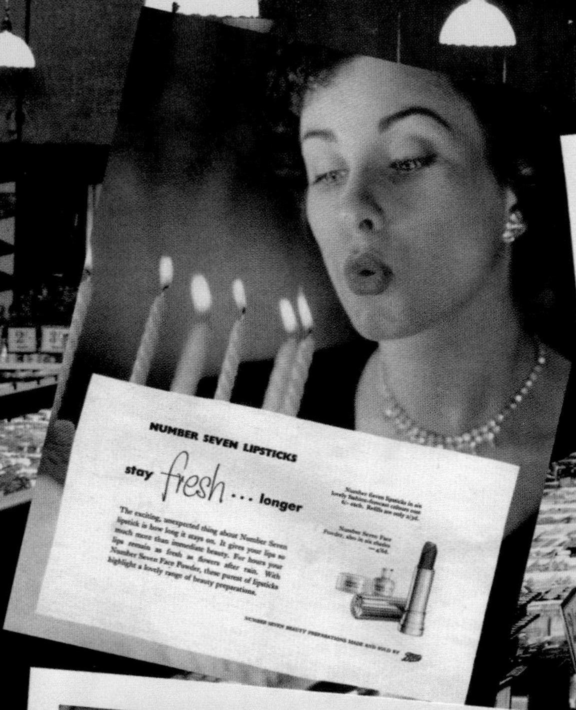

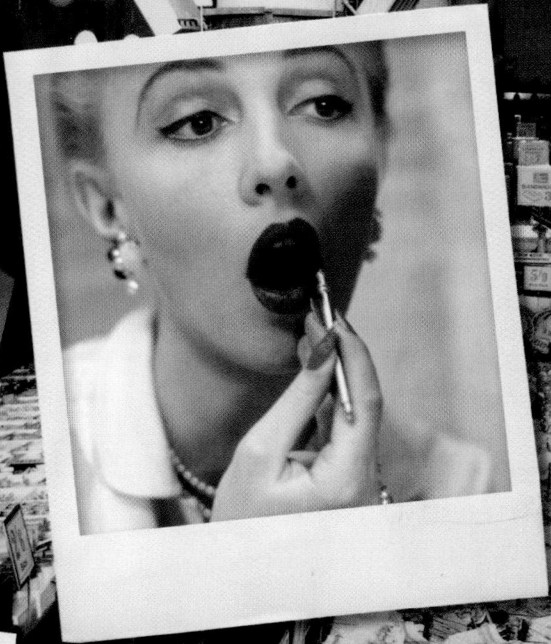

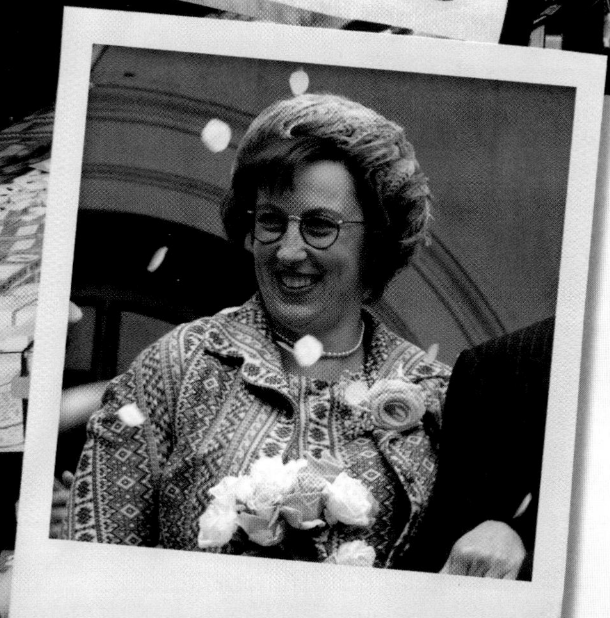

NUMBER SEVEN LIPSTICKS

stay *fresh* ... longer

*Chummy, played by
Miranda Hart, has been
known to splash out in the
lip department, sporting
a slick of bright red on her
wedding day. History failed
to record whether
it was Gay Geranium.*

*In the fifties every woman had a bottle of
Eau de Cologne 4711 somewhere — in the bathroom,
in her handbag, or on a dressing table.*

gangrenous ulcers were created for old soldier Joe Collett, played by Roy Hudd, while Chummy suffered a gravel-pocked graze when she tumbled from her bike. Series Two features an epoch-making chiropody case, as well as cuts and bruises caused by domestic violence.

In the top drawer of my desk, I keep something that not only evokes this common past, but gives me access to it. It is a bottle of Eau de Cologne 4711 – a watery blend of bergamot, citrus, lavender and rosemary. At just a few pounds a pop, it is one of the cheapest perfumes on the market and, dating from 1792, possibly the most enduring. In the fifties, every woman had a bottle somewhere – in the bathroom, in her handbag, or on a dressing table.

'Personal daintiness' was becoming something of a pre-occupation by 1958. Deodorant was in its infancy, talcum powder was popular, and luxury perfumes had started to appear.

There was a talismanic quality to some of these fragrances. *Call the Midwife*'s executive producer Pippa Harris remarks that her mother, Angela, discovered Nina Ricci's L'Air Du Temps as a young woman in the fifties, and went on to wear it all her life. This haunting scent, first launched in 1948, was – and remains – a blend of carnation, rosewood, cedar and iris. 'The bottle had a beautiful glass stopper, styled like two entwined doves,' recalls Pippa. 'But my mother always kept it on her dressing table in its pale yellow carton, to protect the scent from sunlight.'

By 1957, Elizabeth Arden's Blue Grass and Worth's Je Reviens were also in vogue, and the jasmine-heavy Joy held fast to its crown as the world's most costly perfume. But these were all beyond the pockets of working people. For the vast majority of women (and many men), 4711 was the go-to fragrance. It could be splashed on from the bottle or deployed in roll-on form. It cooled and freshened and was reputed to cure headaches. It could be used to scent underclothes and handkerchiefs. It was fresh and ladylike, or manly and respectable. Your mother would have used it, and your mother's mother. It would remind you of people that you loved, just as it reminds me of people I have loved – aunts and grandmas, freshly shaved uncles. Everybody bandbox neat and ready to go out.

Television is not an olfactory medium and I am under no illusion that the *Call the Midwife* cast splash themselves with 4711 before they leave the make-up trailer. But sometimes when I'm tired I take the bottle of cologne out of my desk, rub a little on my wrists and sniff – and I'm right there in Poplar, in 1958. It's the whiff of girls getting ready to go out to a dance, the cooling cloth on the brow of a labouring woman. It's nervous Cynthia fretting about her armpits, Jenny reminded of the man she couldn't have. It is a bridge between that other world and this one, like *Call the Midwife* itself. And I breathe in the scent, and keep on writing.

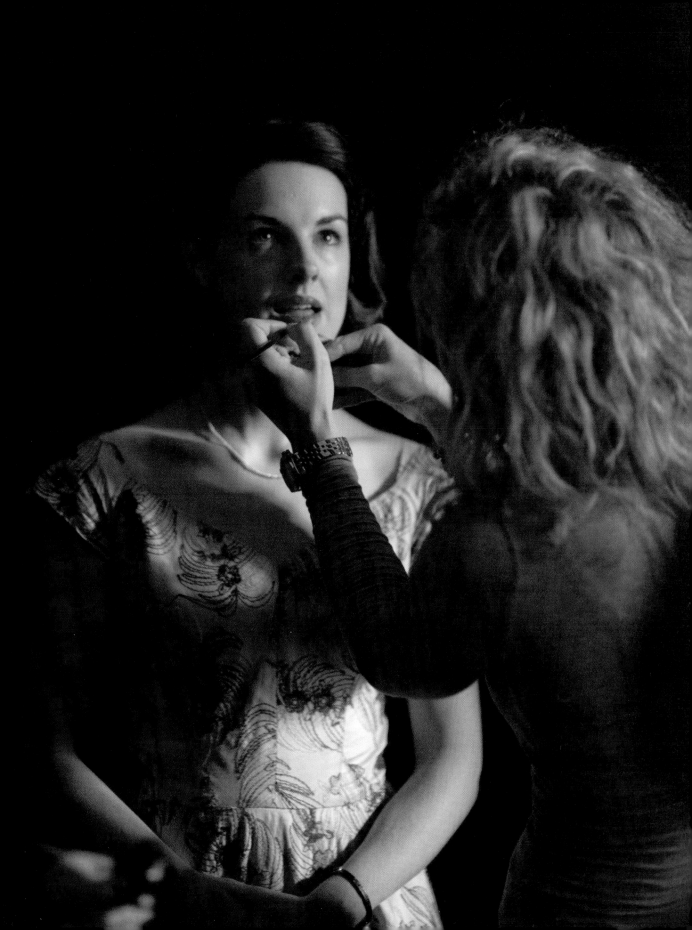

Call the Midwife

Diaries

Part 1

I fall in love with Jennifer Worth's
memoirs, and take quite a shine to
Jennifer herself. But plans for the
series move slowly — we eat cake,
and are frustrated.

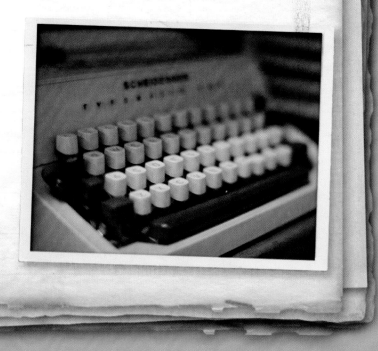

13 May 2008

I have sealed my fate. I have said 'Yes' to turning *Call the Midwife* into a television series. I was so knocked out by my first reading of the book that I e-mailed the Executive Producer, Pippa Harris of Neal Street Productions, in the middle of the night, accepting the commission. Waking this morning, I wonder if I've jumped the gun. This is completely unlike anything I have ever tackled before. Compelling though it is to read, *Call the Midwife* is an odd sort of hybrid; half-novel, half-memoir. The characters are delightful, but some are more fully developed than others, and the East End women speak in a peculiar phonetic dialect of Jennifer Worth's devising. Meanwhile the stories — key to any successful adaptation — are a potentially unfilmable pastiche of obstetrics and social history, with a dash of religion thrown into the mix.

And yet, and yet ... Tears well up again as I remember the story of Conchita Warren, whose premature 25th baby was given up for dead but survived because of her unsparing love. And my lips twitch at the thought of elderly Sister Monica Joan, who reminds me of every bonkers old lady I've ever known (and I've known plenty).

So I do what I always do when my thoughts start swirling — I put my apron on and bake. I am not Saffron Walden's best pâtissière, and I am probably not even its most enthusiastic, but I've never yet turned out a sponge or a tray of scones without feeling better, and more centred. I tell myself that what I will do is get mixing and have a think, and if by the time the cake is cool I still have reservations, I will ring Pippa and pull out of the project.

As I line the tin with greaseproof paper, my mind turns to *Cranford*, the BBC drama series that premiered last winter, but which has, one way or another, dominated the last six years of my life.

Cranford came to me via two gifted women, Sue Birtwistle and Susie Conklin, who had seen the potential in Elizabeth Gaskell's classic but neglected novel, *Cranford*. Like *Call the Midwife*, the original *Cranford* was a memoir fuelled by many years of hindsight. It, too, was a melange of delicious snippets, somewhat untidily gathered, but suffused with warmth and wit. It also had the power to make me weep, yet didn't seem remotely obvious as a candidate for TV adaptation. But in the end, *Cranford* had triumphed.

There is another deep bond between the two books, one I don't consciously notice until I stand in my kitchen weighing out the ingredients for a lavender madeira cake. Cracking the eggs from my sister-in-law Rosie's hens, and sprinkling in the lavender grown by my friend Julie, I realise that what the two books have in common is that they celebrate the lives of women, and the bonds between them. They are set in the past, but concern themselves with pleasures and pains that never change.

Women tell one another stories. It is that simple. It is also that piecemeal, that untidy, that compelling. And we keep on doing it, generation after generation, in letters, in novels, in memoirs, by word of mouth. And on television if (like me, like Pippa) we are daft enough to try.

While the cake rises in the oven, I suddenly feel fiercely protective of Jennifer's work — the frank and magical web of words a woman I've never met wove at her desk, many moons after her retirement from midwifery. I want to play my part in getting those stories out to the wider world, where — if I do my job properly — they will move other women to laughter and to tears.

For the moment, the funniest and saddest thing in my house is the madeira cake. It has stuck to the tin, and I have overdone it with the lavender, so it smells (and will doubtless taste) like the furniture polish my grandma used to like.

But it cools and is eaten anyway, and I never do call Pippa to say I've changed my mind. I am in love with *Call the Midwife*. And that's that.

8 June 2008

I go up to London to meet Jennifer Worth and her husband Philip for lunch with Pippa, who has now commissioned the scripts. We will be joined by Tara Cook, the development executive who first brought the books to Neal Street Production's attention. I feel desperately nervous, change my dress three times, and miss my train, even though I leave the house with my hair still wet.

Train Times

09.30
09.50
10.20

Jennifer and Philip have travelled up from their holiday flat in Brighton, and arrive at the restaurant a little late. They are unmissable as they enter — she tall, dressed in blue and peering politely from her spectacles. He follows a pace or two behind, in a tidy sports coat.

It isn't an interview — I already have the job — but this first encounter feels like a cross between meeting a new headmistress and a blind date that might last several years. Getting a TV show as far as the screen can take a very long time, and it's vital that we get along.

We do get along. I think. The restaurant is wood-panelled and buzzy and the acoustics are abominable. We struggle to converse above the rattle of china and glass. I suspect that, like many people of a certain age, Jennifer may be slightly hard of hearing. When she announces that she turned *Cranford* off after 15 minutes, 'because those Dames have such appalling diction,' this appears to be confirmed.

I mainly chat to Philip, next to whom I have been seated, and he is a delight — very modest and quiet, and extraordinarily proud of Jennifer. He appears to find her late blossoming as an authoress rather startling. Jennifer, one senses, doesn't find it startling at all. This

12.6.08

Dear Pippa,

Thank you so much for a lovely lunch yesterday — we both found it overwhelming but enjoyable; and I look forward to meeting Heidi again in a more working atmosphere.

You asked me about character casting — the girls would be best to be unknown actresses. I am so glad it is mainly female parts, to give young aspirings a chance.

Philip sends his best wishes, and we look forward to meeting again.

Very best wishes
Jennifer Worth

is not because of any arrogance on her part, but because she is a highly accomplished woman who has changed gear often, and with success, throughout her life. After midwifery, she switched to end-of-life care on a Marie Curie cancer ward, then left nursing to pursue a career in music. She excelled in all of these things, as well as in her marriage and as a mother — *Call the Midwife* is simply the icing on the post-retirement cake.

By the time coffee is served, Jennifer and I — by dint of bawling across the table — have made plans to get together some months hence, when I am available to start writing. I find myself fascinated by her long elegant hands, with their large oval rings of opals and sapphires. She is quite unlike anyone I have ever met.

8 January 2009

The plan is to drive to Hemel Hempstead for lunch with Jennifer and Philip, to discuss me starting work on the scripts. It snowed in the night. There are doleful reports on the radio about the state of the M25 and I wonder if we should cancel. But the meeting has been put off before, and Pippa rings to say she is making headway from her home in Oxford, and I crawl all the way, skidding slightly twice in thick brown slush.

I suddenly remember that I turned down a trip to the Golden Globe Awards in order to make this appointment, and feel jealous of my *Cranford* colleagues swanning about in the sunshine of Los Angeles.

I am an hour and a half late, and arrive to find Pippa huddled by the log fire Jennifer has lit in our honour. The house is

Victorian, filled with books and pictures. Philip paints, in the modernist style, and there are quite a lot of portraits of Jennifer. Half the drawing room is taken up with an exquisite antique grand piano, which Jennifer reveals she plays to concert hall standard. In her own home, she seems more authoritative than she did in the restaurant. She can't quite say her 'R's — a fact I didn't notice when we first met — and wears slacks and a tabard. There is a touch of the Queen about her, which I like very much.

Lunch is stew, with an eccentric side dish that Jennifer declares to be her speciality — one large whole onion apiece, wrapped in tinfoil and baked in the oven complete with skin. Unpeeled, they melt into the plate and taste delicious.

Knowing that my work is about to start in earnest, I am brimming with questions, but proceedings are formal and we are on the gooseberry crumble before it feels polite to put her on the spot. Oddly, the thing that breaks the ice is religion. I know from Jennifer's books that she became a committed Christian during her time in the East End. I have always had a religious faith, and though I am now involved with Quakers I was brought up Anglican.

We have a bracing conversation about the Book of Common Prayer, referencing the Evening and Morning Collects, and I mention that my uncle is an Anglican priest. Jennifer seems to like this; religion and spirituality are a very important theme in her

books. Nevertheless, in response to my
polite enquiry, she refuses to reveal
the true identity of the nuns. She says
that when writing the book she changed
their name at their request, and
promised never to reveal it.

By the time I leave, we are inching
towards friendship. She and Philip help me into
my coat, a navy serge number with a voluminous panelled skirt,
which gets them both slightly confused. But when it is on and
buttoned up, Jennifer turns me around and looks at the cut in
an appraising sort of way. 'This reminds me,' she says, 'of a
navy New Look coat I bought in 1958. It had a scarlet lining.'

'I remember that,' says Philip. Jennifer adopts a tone I suspect
I will come to know quite well.

'You must put it in one of your scripts.' And she shows me to
the door.

3 March 2009

Jennifer and I convene again in Hemel Hempstead, this time in
her study. She doesn't call it her study, she calls it The
Blue Room, in honour of the Wedgwood walls. This is where
she wrote *Call the Midwife*, by hand, but there are no books
or papers in it, or even a desk — just a plain table and a
large dark wardrobe with a mirrored door. It is elegant and
somehow Spartan, like Jennifer herself. Downstairs, one of her
granddaughters is having a singing lesson. She is a soprano,
and is working at her scales.

"Let us see what love can do" W. PENN

SR. JULIENNE? or SR M-J

Childrens games

Skipping songs, ball songs, ten pins, marbles, jacks, peg tops, whipping tops, horse chestnuts games, five stones, hoops, lath for rolling and whirling around your waist — great skill required. Diabolo - tossing a huge cotton reel

My imagination feeds on small things, and some days ago, over the phone, I asked Jennifer if she could give me a few more details about life in the East End in the 1950s. She has risen to the challenge with considerable élan, and hands me a dozen sheets of white foolscap, covered in leggy sloping writing. Everything she can remember — but has not mentioned in her books — is there. There is no narrative as such, just a series of lists. But what lists! Children's games, church hall dances, Scout Parades, the scratch of nylons, the taste of Babycham. Jennifer writes with a fountain pen, in soot-coloured ink, which makes the notes feel like a sheaf of black and white photographs, transporting the beholder back to a different time.

One of my main concerns is to find authentic voices for the different groups of characters. The dialogue in the book is not suitable for cutting and pasting into a script (dialogue in books almost never is), and there is a great deal of painstaking work ahead. I quiz Jennifer about the way people spoke. Did they swear? Did they use rhyming slang? Jennifer has very good recall, and I make a lot of notes. When I ask her how the women used to refer to their private parts, she thinks for a moment and says, 'Oh, they used to call it their "downbelows".' I burst out laughing, and so does she. She says it again — 'Downbelows' — in a perfect Cockney accent, as though to reassure herself that that's correct. More laughter. Downstairs, the singing granddaughter hits what sounds like a top B. Jennifer then goes on to cheerfully reveal how women deprived of medical care dealt with prolapse of the womb. The method involved items that could be cheaply purchased at a greengrocer or market stall, and I write it down dutifully, thinking, 'No way is that ever going to make it to the screen.'

23 May 2009

Pippa called two weeks ago, to remind me that the pilot script for *Call the Midwife* is well overdue. In addition to writing the opening episode, I have committed to creating a series 'bible' involving eight separate storylines and character breakdowns for all of our main players. It is intricate work, not helped by the fact that my diary is a shambles.

The sequel to *Cranford* is about to start filming at London's Ealing Studios, and my theatre play about the Russian Revolution, *The House of Special Purpose*, has begun rehearsals in a hall near Chelsea Bridge. Torn three ways, I've booked myself into a hotel in Chiswick, attending two sets of rehearsals during the day and sitting up all night every night writing *Call the Midwife*.

The director of *Cranford*, Simon Curtis, has bought me a chocolate owl as a good luck present. I mean to keep it as a souvenir, but today, at 5am — with the finish line in sight - I capitulate and eat it, ears first. I complete the script at 6.30am, e-mail it to Pippa, sleep for 50 minutes, and go to watch rehearsals for my play.

By lunchtime, the Romanovs have all been shot and Pippa has texted me: 'Top work, Miss Thomas!' I would like to say I burst into tears of happiness, but I just wander down to Cheyne Walk and lie on a bench like a tramp.

18 June 2009

With Pippa's guidance, I have polished Episode One and Jennifer has now read it. Instead of giving her notes over the telephone, or setting them down in a letter, she has written them all over the script and sent it back by return of post. Most of the notes are quite difficult to decipher, since she has been puzzled by the story order, and made a lot of observations that she then went back to cross out, or contradict. She has also amended a lot of the dialogue, so that all the Cockneys drop their aitches and say things like 'Oo' instead of 'Who', just as they do in the book.

LILIAN (CONT'D)
She can't get a man of her own, that's her trouble.

SISTER EVANGELINA
I came here to assess you for a home delivery, not to discuss your neighbour's love-life.

LILIAN
I've had both my other two at home, no trouble. You know that.

SISTER EVANGELINA pours tea into two tin mugs.

LILIAN (CONT'D)
You ought to put yours in a cup and saucer.

SISTER BERNADETTE
I don't want to disturb your sideboard.

But the interesting thing is that as Jennifer works her way through the episode she clearly gets to grips with the way a script is structured, and stops resisting the changes we have made. The notes peter out well before the closing page. There are only two comments that make the final cut, and she sums them up in her covering letter:

(1) Why is it a coconut cake? I did not specify what type of cake it was in the book.

(2) You describe Jenny as arriving in a houndstooth suit. I think she should be in a navy coat with a scarlet lining.

But then she closes with the words, 'If you carry on like this you are going to be up for another BAFTA.' And I heave a sigh of relief.

28 October 2009

It is five months since the BBC took delivery of the first script and the bible for *Call the Midwife*. It was received enthusiastically, but since then the trail has gone cool rather fast. Pippa has worked hard to try to move things on, but we are beginning to feel despondent.

We arrange to meet Jennifer and Philip for tea at Fortnum and Mason, as much to cheer ourselves up as anything else. There is a dull ache about proceedings at the moment. We keep the faith, and a cheerful countenance, but *Call the Midwife* seems to be slipping from our grasp.

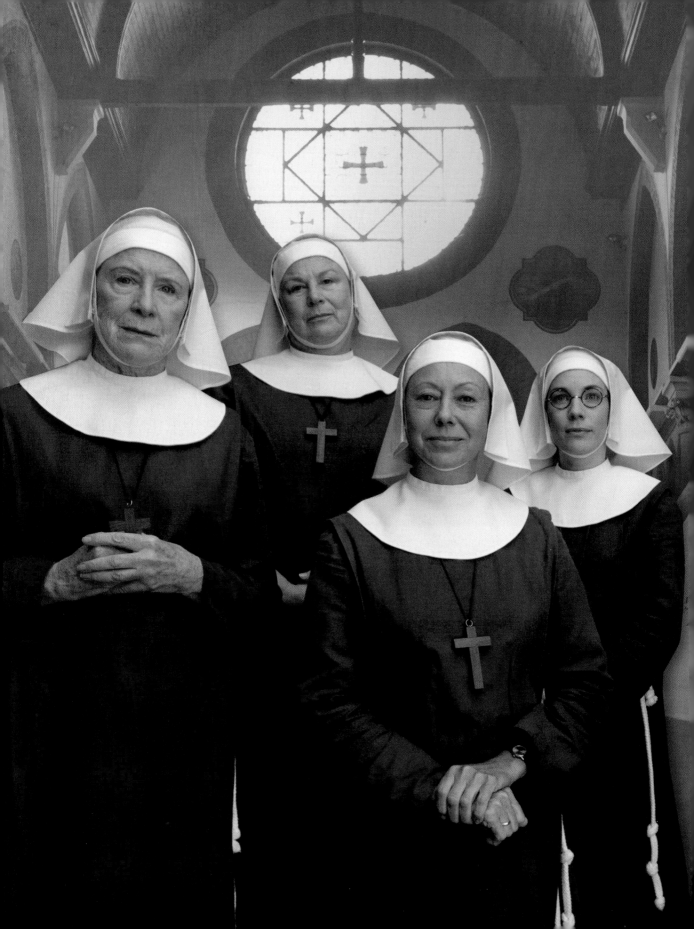

CHAPTER

4

FAITH

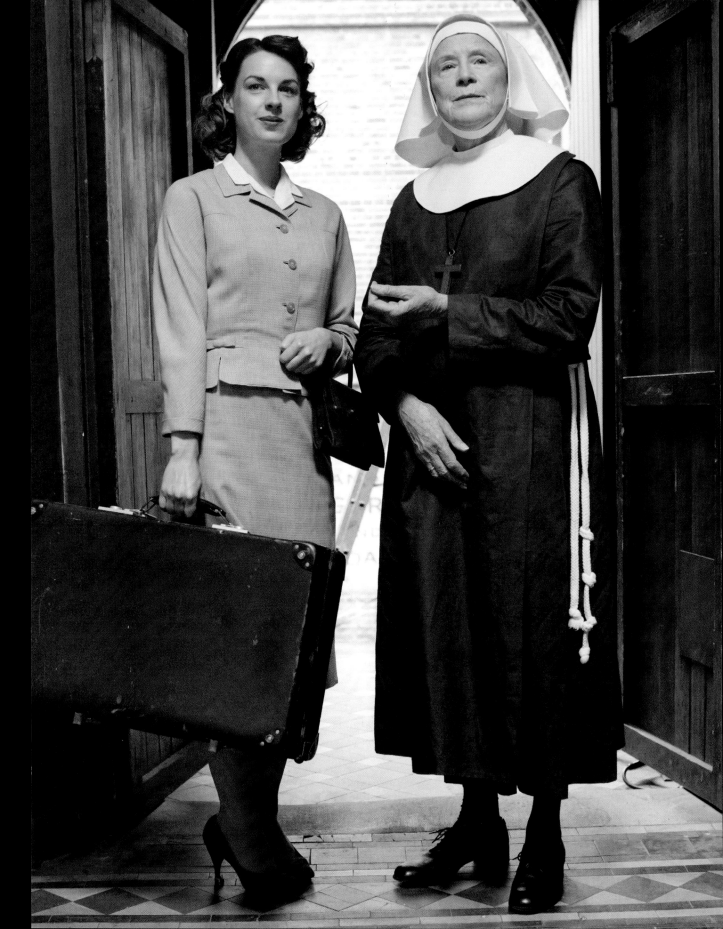

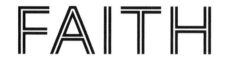

FAITH

'DO YOU HAVE A FAITH, NURSE LEE?'
SISTER JULIENNE

'NOT REALLY. I'M CHURCH OF ENGLAND.'
JENNY

In the opening episode of *Call the Midwife*, young nurse Jenny Lee receives a stark introduction to life in Poplar. After witnessing a street fight, a stained mattress, and domestic overcrowding, she is finally undone by an encounter with a patient in the clinic. After Pearl Winston, heavily pregnant, climbs up on the couch, announcing 'I've got some shocking discharge', Jenny discovers symptoms of advanced venereal disease. Shaking with shock, as she scrubs her hands clean, Jenny says to Sister Julienne 'I didn't know people lived like this.' And Sister Julienne replies, with devastating simplicity, 'But they do. And it's why we're here.'

There could be no clearer way of summing up the Sisters' mission. The fictional Order of St Raymond Nonnatus is inspired by the real life Community of St John the Divine, whose Sisters lived in Poplar for many decades, working amongst the very poorest and most needy.

In the series, we wanted to show how vital the nuns' work was in a challenging and changing world. They are never morally permissive, but nor are they judgemental. In Episode Five of Series One, Jenny is shocked to discover that a middle-aged brother and sister, Frank and Peggy, are living together as man and wife. Sister Evangelina and Sister Julienne simply turn a calm, blind eye to the matter. They are aware of the siblings' appalling, loveless childhood in the workhouse, and see the incest as a direct result of this. This response is inspired by Christian love.

The modern day Community of St John the Divine, just seven in number, are based in urban Birmingham. They are no longer engaged in nursing or midwifery, but exist to promote 'all aspects of health, healing, pastoral care, and

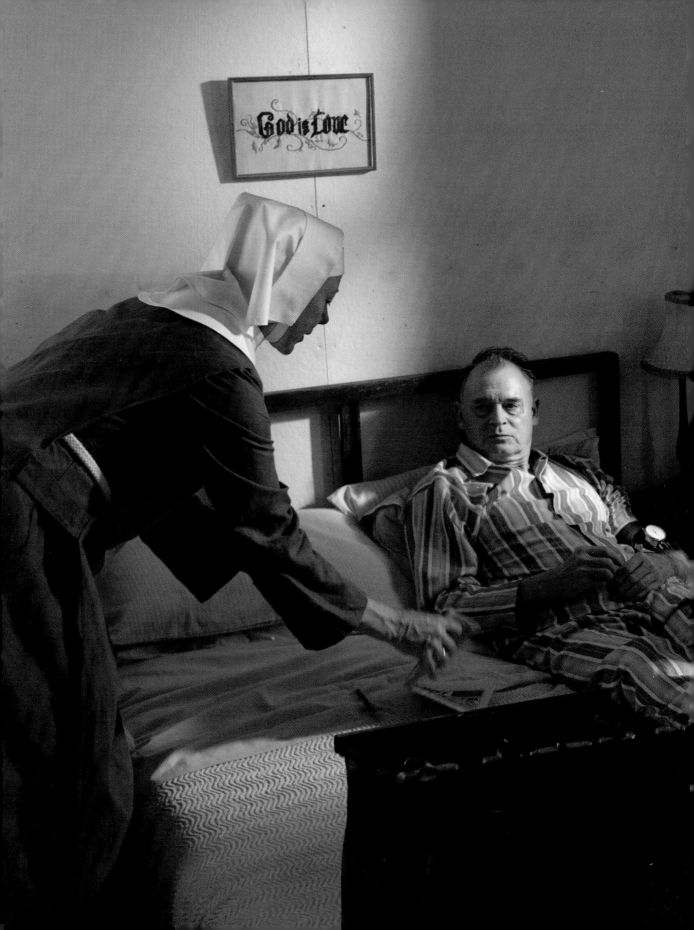

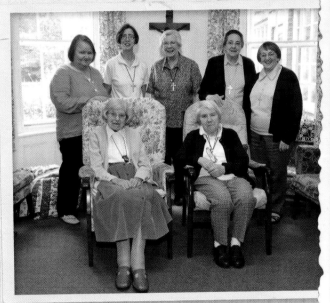

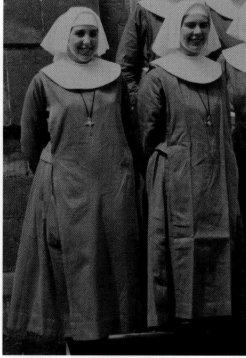

The Community of St John the Divine, who inspired the fictional Order of St Raymond of Nonnatus.

Sister Christine and Sister Margaret-Angela of the Community of St John the Divine, in Poplar in the 1960s.

reconciliation in its widest context.' The fact that this information is summed up on their website says much about the way they move with the times. Yet for Sisters Teresa, Margaret-Angela, Ivy, Shirley, Ruth, Elaine and Christine, their Christian faith is still at the heart of all they do.

Perhaps the most striking thing about a day spent with the Sisters is how seldom – outside chapel – God or Christ are mentioned. There is no preaching, no rhetoric, no quoting from the Gospels. Each has a heavy silver cross about her neck, but they wear no habit, and dress in a very ordinary way. Nevertheless, any visitor cannot escape the sense that this is a special place, and they are not like other women. Gradually, I realise that they do not need to speak of their

faith, because they embody it. Their beliefs are not boasted of, but lived.

The nuns describe themselves as having a 'ministry of hospitality', and no one in need of nourishment or care is turned away. Homeless men who appear on the doorstep – whom they respectfully refer to as 'our wayfarers' – are provided with a hot drink and sandwiches, and they occasionally give refuge to those suffering from domestic violence or abuse. This is all offered up in a completely loving and accepting way. Sister Christine, who was a midwife in Poplar in the early sixties explains their non-judgemental stance thus: 'From the very beginning, we have been in the middle of real life, and worked with people on the margins of society.'

Jenny Agutter (Sister Julienne) with Sean Baker, who played Frank in Episode Five.

The Community began life in the 1840s, as a training school for nurses working with the London poor. By the 1920s they were completely dedicated to the service of the people of Deptford and Poplar. Their commitment to midwifery increased, and they finally became a formal religious order, with the Sisters taking vows of poverty, chastity and obedience.

In the fifties there was still extraordinary hardship in the homes they visited. Bathrooms were not common, and in some Victorian tenements several families shared a lavatory. Properties waiting to be demolished were frequently verminous, with colonies of bugs entrenched behind decaying plaster. These homes were often inhabited by the elderly, and their stoical endurance was illustrated by the story of old Joe Collet (below), played by Roy Hudd in Series One. His home, scheduled for demolition, was filthy. When Jenny complains about the lack of hygiene, Sister Julienne is uncharacteristically sharp. 'Your comfort is not important,' she tells the young nurse. 'You have a job to do, and you will do it.'

During their decades in Poplar, the nuns strove to balance the demands of the medical and the spiritual, the sacred and profane, the commonplace and the miraculous. At a time when single mothers were reviled, they tended them with the same respect and consideration as the married. In addition, they made no distinction between patients of one faith and another. Whatever the race or creed of a patient, she was there to be served, and serve they did. This lack of prejudice cut two ways, and they were welcomed into homes where the door was barred to others.

The whole *Call the Midwife* team was, from the very outset, anxious to get the portrayal of

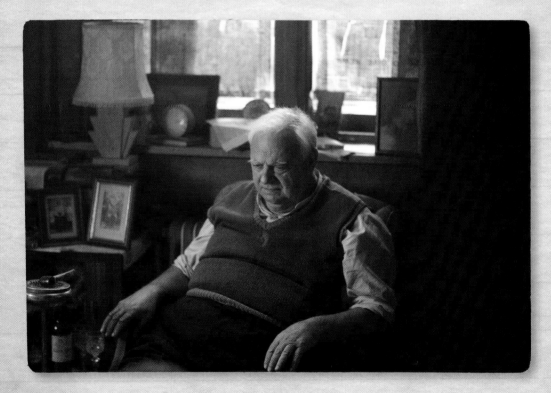

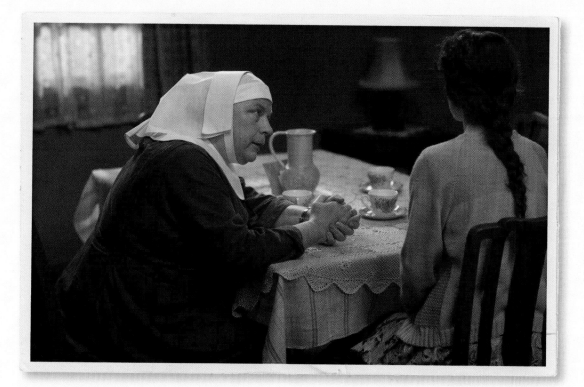

this rare female outfit absolutely right. We were not helped, initially, by Jennifer's refusal to tell us who they were. When she had first shown us the real-life community an early draft of her *Call the Midwife* book, they enjoyed it, but expressed concerns. It contained certain inventions, which, though delightful, to their minds made the book slightly more fiction than fact. Jennifer, who had remained close to the Community, immediately agreed to change various details, concealing their identity.

After a few trips to the archives – and some consultation with my uncle, a priest – we came up with the name of the Order of St John the Divine. Everything fitted, and – when gently pressed – Jennifer came clean, even seeming a bit relieved. Pippa immediately made contact with Sister Christine, and engineered a very happy collaboration with the Community.

Call the Midwife's lead director, Philippa Lowthorpe, sums up the television version of the nuns. 'Our approach to faith was clear eyed, unsentimental and respectful. I'm not a religious person but it was really important to respect that aspect. You have got to see them not only as nuns and midwives but as women, going out into the world and dealing with difficult situations with such aplomb.'

Their work was relentless. All Saints' Church also employed parish workers, either curates or licensed lay people, who were known to go out after breakfast and not return until dark. Sister Margaret-Angela, now in her seventies, began her own life in Poplar in this role. She soon felt called to the religious life, and joined the Sisters in the early sixties. Another notable parish worker – who, though deeply faithful, never took holy vows – was Daphne Jones.

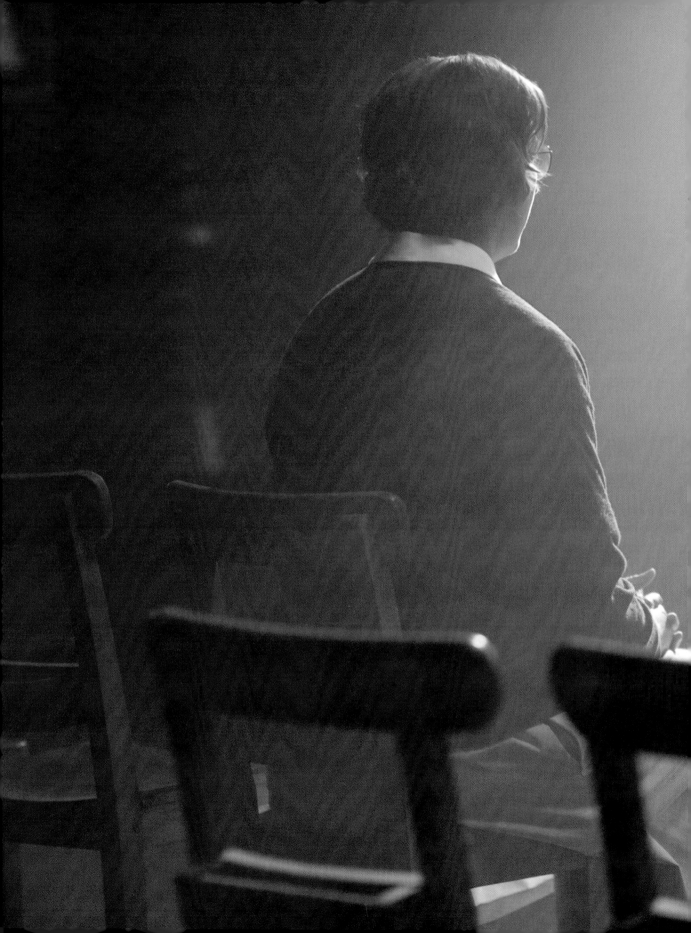

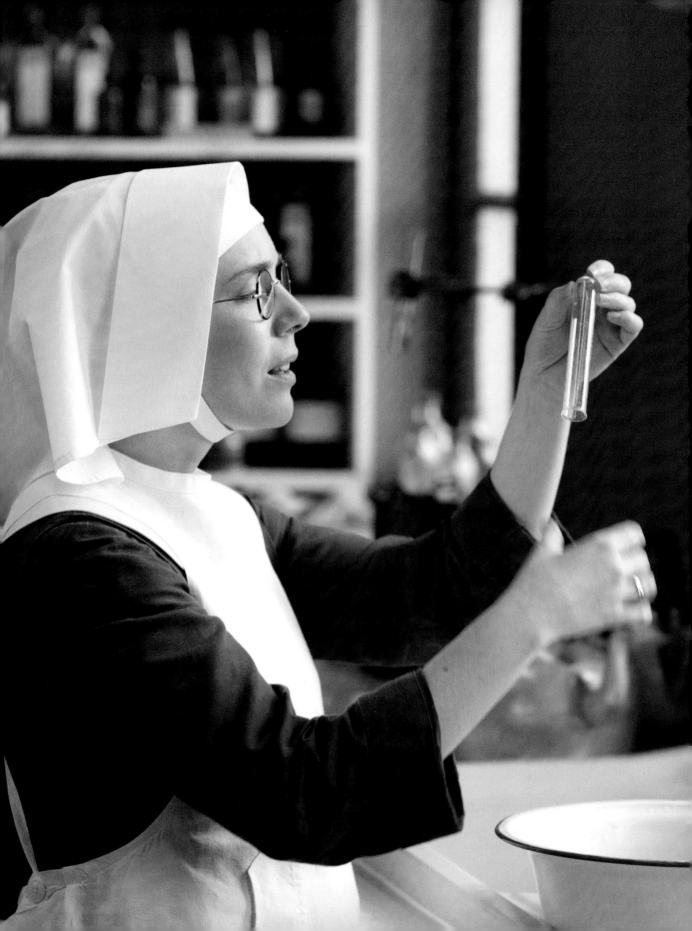

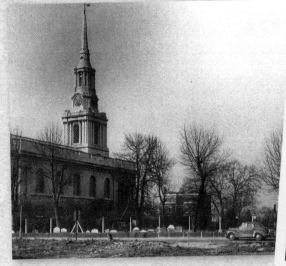

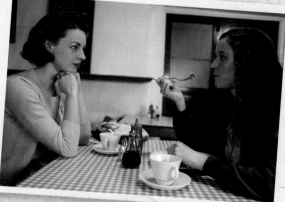

All Saints' Parish Church, Poplar, in 1956.

Born into a wealthy Gloucestershire family in 1915, she was to notch up an incredible 55 years as an All Saints parish worker, working with alcoholics, itinerants, poor families and the sick.

Daphne was a compelling storyteller. In one interview, she described the hazards of being a Poplar parish worker, remembering amongst other things, '... the night Tony from the Vaseline factory came in dead drunk wielding a carving knife.' This did not intimidate Daphne, 'I've always reckoned you can push drunks over.'

One of Daphne's own experiences – that of meeting a teenage Irish prostitute – was picked up by Jennifer and incorporated into her memoirs. In turn, the story of 'Mary' was featured in the series. It is a harrowing account of a vulnerable child tricked into a life in the sex trade, where unwanted pregnancy could lead to enforced, illegal abortion or even death. Once rescued, all the care Mary receives is connected

> ## All the care Mary receives is connected in some way with religious organisations.

in some way with religious organisations. She is taken in first by Sister Julienne, then by a women's refuge run by a priest, Father Joe, and is ultimately sent to a Catholic mother and baby home. This care is never judgemental, and always compassionate, but when Mary's weeks-old daughter is taken from her, her grief is extreme. Father Joe's response is impassioned: 'How can a 15-year-old girl with no education, no home, and no way of earning a living other than through the trade of prostitution take care of a baby?', he asks a furious Jenny. 'It was a question of which child should we choose!'

Dilemmas such as this were part and parcel of work amongst society's most needy.

The Community of St John the Divine left Poplar in 1978, ostensibly because of a rent hike, but in reality, their work in the district had been completed. At the time that *Call the Midwife* is set, each midwife at Nonnatus House could expect to attend three deliveries each week – but massive change was just around the corner.

In Series One of *Call the Midwife* Sister Evangelina – cycling vigorously down a side street – observes, 'There are between eighty and one hundred births each month in Poplar. As soon as one vacates the pram, another one takes its place. And thus it was and ever shall be, until they invent a magic position that will put a stop to it'.

That is exactly what happened. The contraceptive pill was first made available in 1961, through family planning clinics. Combined with a burgeoning move towards hospital delivery it gradually put the bicycling midwives out of business. Initially, the Sisters still worked in the district. But they were deployed as staff members at NHS clinics, and lost a degree of autonomy. Also, local authorities were not always at ease having nuns on the premises. As Sister Margaret-Angela remarks, 'We did get quite a few looks going into the family planning clinic.' Sister Christine continued to work as a midwife tutor for some years, but developed reservations about the changes in midwifery education. She strongly believed that people not wishing to study to degree level could make wonderful midwives, but the emphasis was increasingly on classroom study, and nursing degrees became the norm. Sister Christine realised that her vocation was changing, and embarked on a period of prayer and reflection. Unsurprisingly, this didn't involve much sitting down.

'I took time out. I spent eighteen months in the Community's five-storey house in Vauxhall. Every day I scrubbed the walls, the paintwork and the carpet, praying about what I should do. There was no clear answer. I missed midwifery so much, but then came the awareness that I was being asked to put down midwifery. Eventually, after many tears, I realised that God was helping me to understand that I could still be a midwife, but in a different way.'

As a result of this revelation Sister Christine no longer delivers babies, but devotes herself to supporting others at times of spiritual – rather than physical – duress. 'Spiritual accompaniment' is now part of the Sisters' mission.

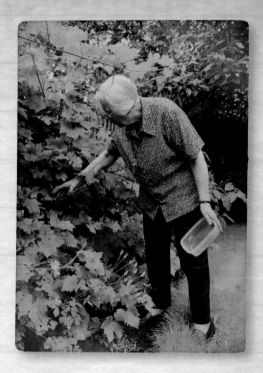

Sister Margaret-Angela of the Community of St John the Divine, picking berries in the convent garden.

The Community of St John the Divine's buildings are used as a centre of prayer by the diocese of Birmingham. Rooms are available for quiet days and meetings, and the nuns are active in community affairs, seeking constantly to build bridges and mend lives. But the convent is perhaps, above all else, an inspiring and happy home, where all who enter are made welcome. Sisters Ivy and Sister Elaine command the kichen, offering magnificent cooked lunches. Elaine is also a reflexologist. The nuns grow their own vegetables and fruit, bake their own bread and make jam.

It is a small but vibrant community, that has passed through changing times, emerging quietly triumphant. There is no longer an elected 'mother Superior'; leadership is shared, and based on consultation. Everything is debated, and nothing rushed into, for they are

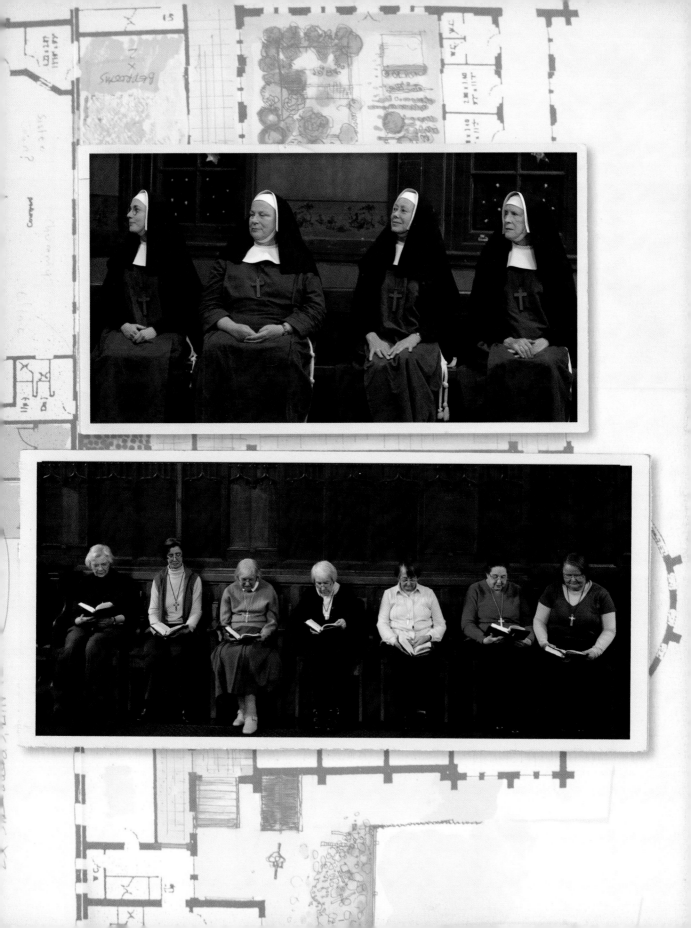

conscious that the Community has a rich history, throughout which much has been accomplished. 'We want to make sure we don't throw the baby out with the bathwater,' explains Sister Christine.

As testament to this, the last habit and wimple belonging to the Community are now tucked up in a drawer. In the eighties, a holiday spent climbing in the Lake District in shin-length habits convinced them to drop the 'uniform' when they weren't at work. Soon afterwards – as always, after a period of prayer and reflection – the community adopted informal dress across the board.

And so the nuns keep moving forward. But, sometimes, it seems as though the world is moving faster. Over the last fifty years, fewer young people have felt the call to the religious life. Like other Orders, the Community of St John the Divine had dwindled dramatically in size. Only one new member, Sister Ruth, has joined in recent years. In order to cope with this trend, the Anglican church has considered opening up new models for religious life – for example, allowing a finite commitment for a two to five year period. But for the truly faithful, there has always been a way.

Some of the most moving and beautifully filmed sequences in *Call the Midwife* depict the nuns in the act of worship. In almost every episode, we hear their voices raised in praise and see their work-worn hands wrapped around blue prayer books. These are originals, used in the

fifties, a gift to the show from the Sisters themselves. I keep a copy on my desk, and on the first faded page is the inscription, 'In the evening, and morning, and at noonday I will pray to thee.'

Hugh Warren, the producer, was at first slightly worried about whether this material would work. 'I am a firm atheist in the Dawkins school,' he reveals, 'I was very nervous about the nuns singing, as I thought it could be a real turn off for a non-religious audience. But I underestimated the power of the human voice.

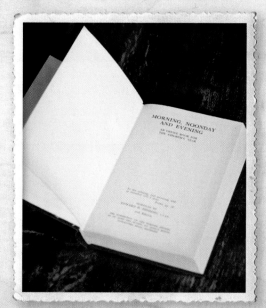

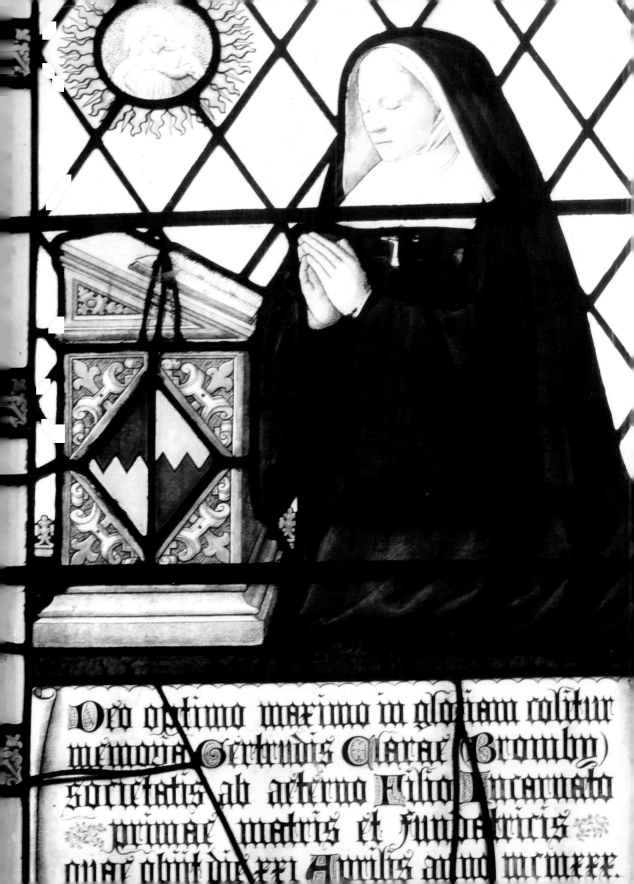

Deo optimo maximo in gloriam colitur
memoria Gertrudis Clarae (Bromby)
societatis ab aeterno Filio Incarnato
primae matris et fundatricis
qua obiit die xxi Aprilis anno domini mcmxxx

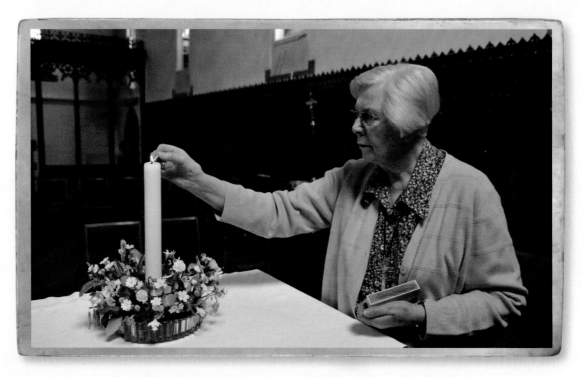

Sister Margaret-Angela lighting the Paschal candle, which is adorned with a delicate garland of Sister Ivy's sugarcraft flowers.

Why I don't know, as the singing at Welsh rugby matches and Thomas Tallis's *Spem in Alium* always reduce me to tears. In the end, I found these scenes extraordinarily affecting and powerful, and they spoke of respect and love, not proselytising.'

In 2012, the days of the Sisters still pivot around prayer. This begins at 6.30am. They pray in silence, often using candles or flowers as a focus, intent upon their own devotions. An hour later Morning Prayer – a spoken service – begins. The remainder of the day is taken up with meetings, meals and other busy interactions, but is structured around religious activity. A visiting priest will conduct the Eucharist at 12.30pm, Evening Prayer is at 5pm and Compline is at 8pm. After Compline, the Sisters are silent until the following morning. They describe this as anchoring and restorative, a uniform, perfect end to their busy and varied days.

All worship takes place in the beautiful Edwardian chapel, linked to the convent by a cloistered way. When refurbishments were required some years ago Sister Ivy – then in her sixties – undertook a sponsored sky dive to raise funds. 'She was strapped to a very handsome young man,' observes Sister Christine, 'and raised £8,000.' In press pictures of the jump, helmeted Sister Ivy is clearly wearing her trusty silver cross.

That same cross is in evidence in a local cake-shop twice a week, where skilled pâtissière Ivy has a part-time job. This simple commitment is perceived as a ministry, making faith visible in a troubled world. At the other end of the scale, her sugar craft skills create exquisite decorations for the convent chapel. An Easter garland of fondant flowers, designed to collar the Paschal candle, is breathtaking in its beauty. To me, this ornament sums up the Sisters' way of life – ordinary, humble ingredients, worked into a glorious offering to God.

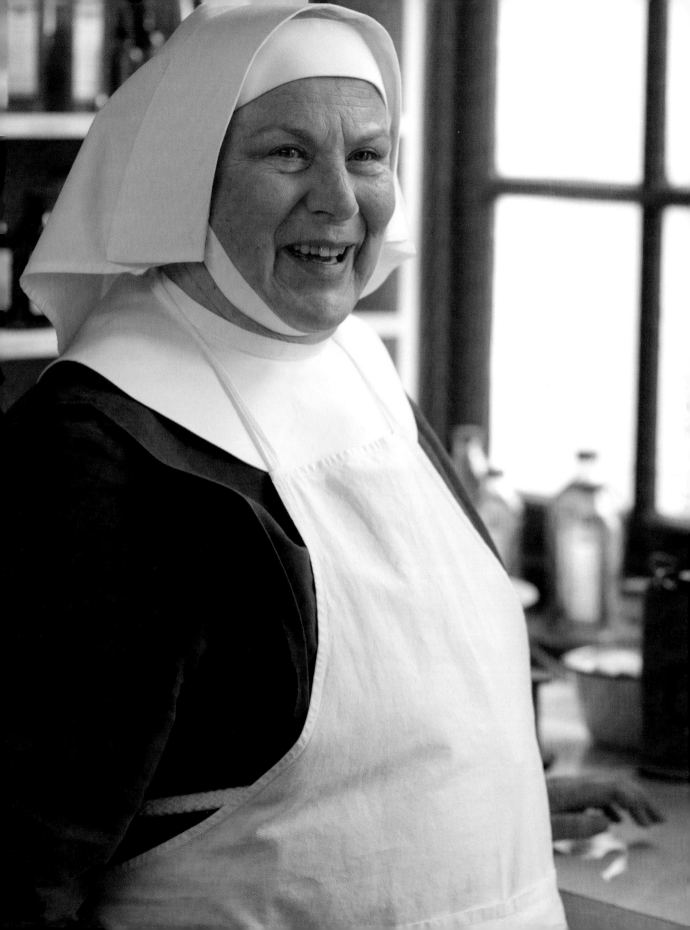

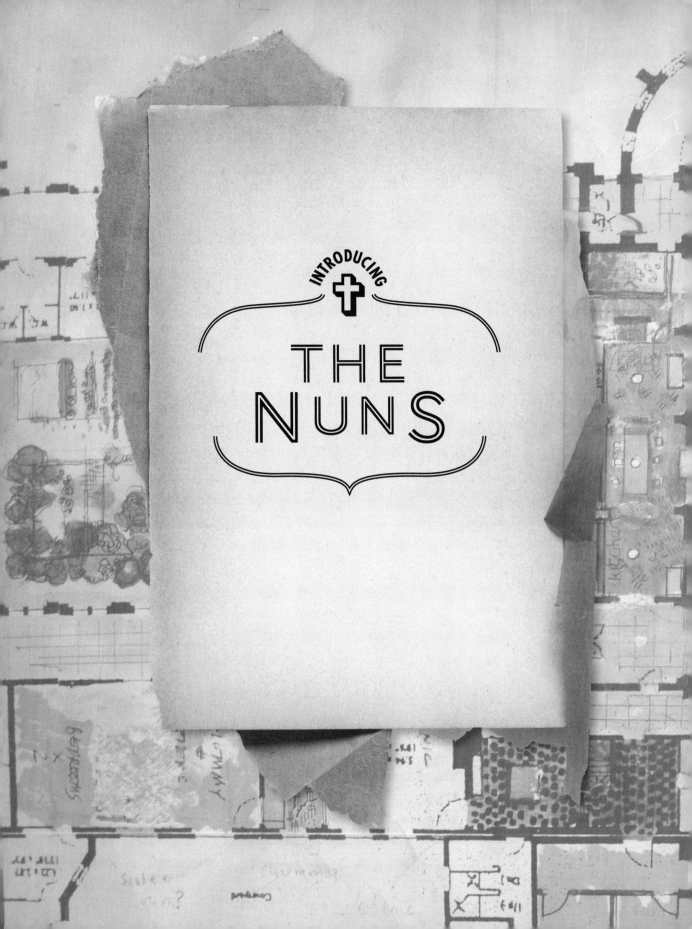

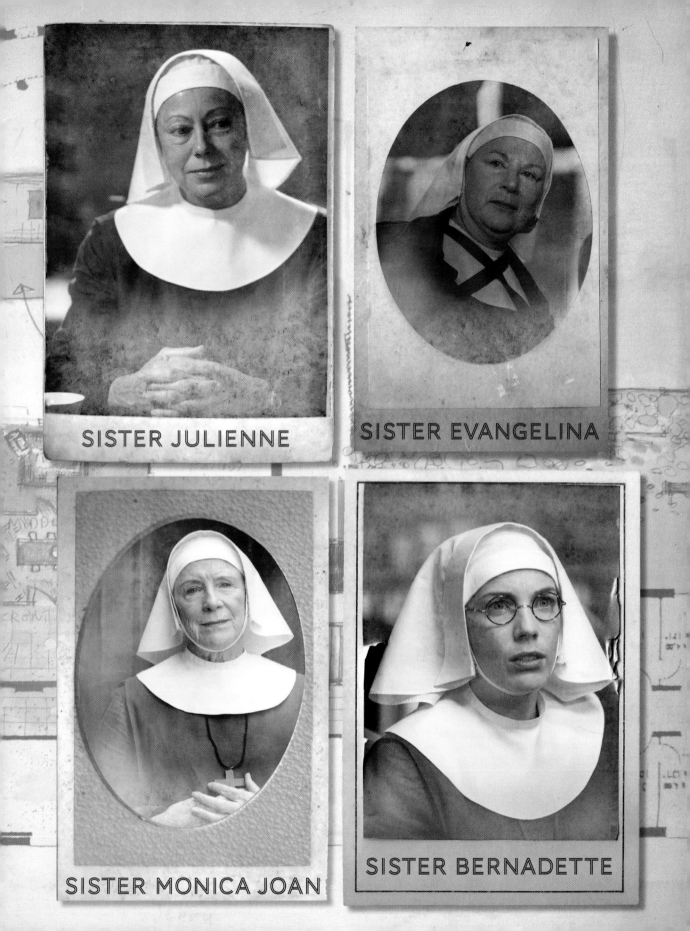

SISTER JULIENNE

SISTER EVANGELINA

SISTER MONICA JOAN

SISTER BERNADETTE

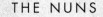

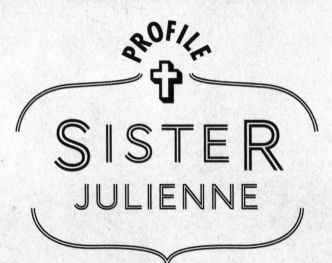

PROFILE
✟
SISTER
JULIENNE

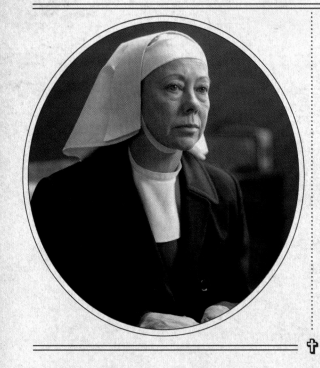

Sister Julienne was an intriguing personality to transfer to the screen. Jennifer Worth had a gift for sustaining friendships over long periods of time, but her connection with the real-life 'Julienne' was notably deep and clearly special to them both.

As I gained Jennifer's trust, I gathered from our conversations that the character in the books was based on a certain Sister Jocelyn of the Order of St John the Divine.

It seemed to me that her key attributes were sincerity and charm, and these were a pleasure to put onto the page. But once the scripts were written we had to find the actress who could play her. *Call the Midwife*'s brilliant casting director, Andy Pryor, knew the answer in a moment. 'Jenny Agutter,' he said. An established star since her teens, Jenny has grace, poise and good humour in abundance. And, as a gentleman of my

✟

acquaintance once remarked, she's got 'the sort of face you'd like to see when you're coming round from an anaesthetic'.

Catholic by upbringing and spiritual by nature, Jenny can identify with much that she sees in Sister Julienne. 'She's responsible and in charge, but there's a twinkle there and a sense of fun. Nothing is mundane, life is amazing.'

When I was working on the scripts, I had no contact with Sister Jocelyn's family. Sister Julienne was at least partly a creation of Jennifer's imagination and, like all good writers, she had nipped and tucked the truth in order to protect her subject and create a more satisfying whole. Nevertheless, further down the line, Jenny Agutter enjoyed a fruitful correspondence with Sister Jocelyn's surviving family. To her surprise, Jenny discovered that the Sister, troubled about the change in Sunday trading laws, once tackled Prime Minister Margaret Thatcher.

'For her, Sunday was a day of rest and was not intended for working. She clearly felt strongly about certain issues and set about them in her own quiet way.'

However, there comes a point where Jenny parts company with the character she plays.

'There's sometimes an acceptance in her that I don't fully understand,' she admits. 'Julienne has absolute faith, and is motivated by her sense of service to people. She doesn't have a critical eye. For her the whole point is to take care of things the way God has made it. She just deals with what is there, and believes that everything is redeemable.'

Jenny herself is too spirited to accept some of the shocking situations she encounters, and she has channelled this energy for change into charity work. She supports numerous good causes, including Action for Children and the ovarian cancer fund

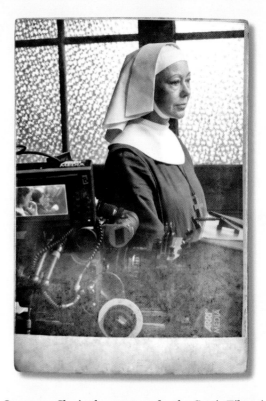

Ovacome. She is also a patron for the Cystic Fibrosis Trust and CHICKS, which provides breaks for hard-pressed children. In addition, she is involved with the St Giles Trust, which helps ex-offenders and other disadvantaged people. In recognition of this work, Jenny was awarded an OBE in the Jubilee year's Queen's birthday honours list. She said it was a humbling experience.

'I have worked very closely with these organisations, and I'm the person at the front getting the attention. But there are so many other people lined up behind me who carry out work day to day for these charities, many of them volunteers. Charities could not work without people like that behind them. If this helps to shine the spotlight on them, then I'm delighted.'

Meanwhile, Jenny is still digesting the overwhelming success of the *Call the Midwife* series. She believes that much of the power of the series lies in its essential optimism. 'Birth itself is about rejuvenation, hope, and all the possibilities that lie ahead.'

Q&A

What are the best things about being a nun?
The sense of community amongst the sisters, and – at night – the privilege of silence.

Is there anything you miss since taking your vows?
My family. I am not forbidden to see them, but the level of commitment to our nursing work makes visits few and far between.

If you could take a holiday, where would you go?
The Scilly Isles. The wide open skies and the lack of traffic would be manna for the soul.

Do you have a favourite piece of music or book (apart from the Bible)?
As a child, I read *What Katy Did* a dozen times. Perhaps it says something to me about the power of the human spirit, but I reach for it like a comfort blanket whenever times are hard.

Do you have time for hobbies?
The Sisters have an hour of recreation each day, although we're often too busy to take a break at all! I enjoy working with water-colours, and always paint my Christmas cards by hand.

What's your favourite smell?
Lilac, after it has rained. I know every lilac tree in Poplar – there aren't that many! – and after a heavy shower I've been known to take a detour on my bicycle, just to enjoy the perfume.

What's your most treasured memory?
The first baby I delivered; a little boy with ginger hair. I can remember cutting the cord as though it happened yesterday.

What's your secret vice?
Custard. I have been known to have second helpings.

And your dearest wish?
To see the National Health Service go from strength to strength.

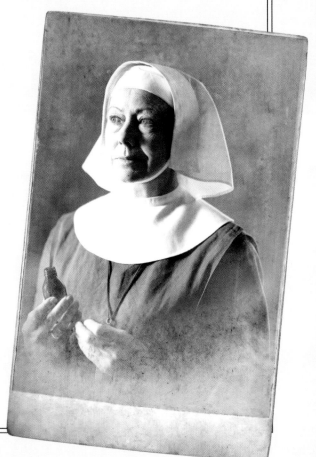

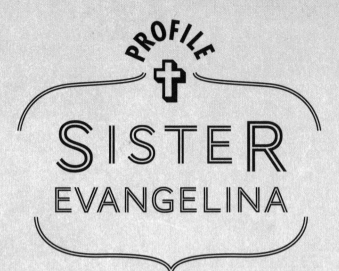

PROFILE

SISTER EVANGELINA

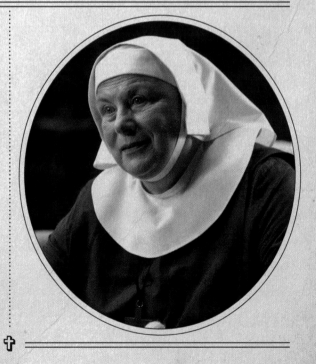

For Pam Ferris, *Call the Midwife* marks the second time she has made an onscreen return to the fifties and found herself in a hit.

She starred as Ma Larkin in ITV's *The Darling Buds of May*, screened in the early nineties. Light-hearted, sensuous Ma could hardly be further from plain-speaking Sister Evangelina, but Pam thrives on contrasting roles. 'I first heard about *Call the Midwife* a few days before I was sent the script and I thought, "That sounds right up my street."'

Pam accepted the offer of the role at once and has huge admiration for the woman she portrays. 'Sister Evangelina is able to talk to people around the East End in their own language. That is a terrific quality,' says Pam. 'She is utterly dedicated to the community she works for, and she never lets up.'

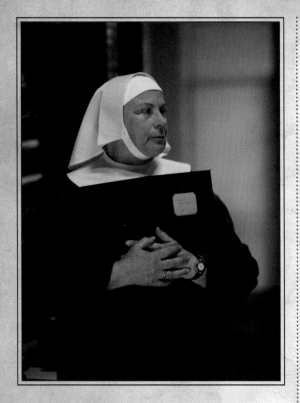

'Sister Evangelina is able
to talk to people around
the East End in their own
language.'

PAM FERRIS

✝

The sister's humble beginnings have influenced the way Pam has chosen to portray the character. 'She was probably brought up in a poor household. Her table manners aren't always great. But she also eats quickly because she doesn't want to waste time – she could be spending that time looking after her patients. There is a driven quality to Evangelina, and I felt she would move fast in whatever she does.'

Small details like this are, to Pam, the foundation of a good performance. 'You make certain decisions about a character, about where she comes from, why she is dedicated in the way she is – and in the end, it should look completely obvious.'

Pam, a stickler for research, once vetoed one of her own ideas. Drawing on her own memories of fifties' television, she recalled an advertisement for toilet soap that featured model Katie Boyle. 'It goes, "You will be a little lovelier each day, with fabulous pink Camay",' laughs Pam. 'I had thought I might be able to sing it to a patient – I even rehearsed it!'

But she suddenly realised that the sisters of Nonnatus House would not have had a television set and so know nothing of commercial breaks. She scrapped the idea. 'If you create a world, you cannot break the rules of it,' she says.

Pam applies the same standards to others. When a disgruntled viewer wrote to the *Radio Times* complaining that our midwives measured bumps in centimetres, Pam took up the cudgels and wrote back. She corrected this error in no uncertain terms – by the fifties, midwives were using both Imperial and metric, and we had the books to prove it on the show. The letter was published, alongside a picture of Pam looking ever so slightly truculent, in costume.

Sister Evangelina would be proud.

Q&A

What are the best things about being a nun?
Comfortable shoes and a sense of purpose. I'm not going to discuss my relationship with the Almighty. That's between me and Him.

Is there anything you miss since taking your vows?
When I was growing up, we always had a terrier of some sort, generally with a bit of Westie in the mix. There's something about a dog's head on your knee when you sit down at the end of a busy day. I miss that.

If you could take a holiday, where would you go?
The Mother House in Chichester would do me fine. The meals are reliable and there are some bracing walks.

Do you have a favourite piece of music or book (apart from the Bible)?
I know every word to 'Tomorrow Is A Lovely Day' by Vera Lynn. We used to sing it during the Blitz, when everyone was sleeping in the Tube. We never knew what we'd find when the bombs stopped falling and we came out from underground – but I sometimes think that song gave us the courage to keep going.

Do you have time for hobbies?
No.

What's your favourite smell?
I think pine disinfectant is very underrated. If I go into a patient's home and get a whiff of that, I can be sure I'm in a well-ordered dwelling. People say cleanliness is next to Godliness, but when it comes to midwifery, cleanliness wins hands down.

What's your most treasured memory?
A few days before I joined the Order as a postulant, I helped my parents move to their new council house. They'd raised a family of eight in two rooms, and never had running water indoors before. Here, they had a gas fire and a proper bathroom. I felt I could turn to my vocation, content that they were in a decent place at last.

What's your secret vice?
I'm a bit too fond of heavyweight boxing. When there's a match on the radio, I fill all the moves in in my head. It can get quite savage.

And your dearest wish?
That one day men will stop seeing the contraceptive sheath as an affront to their masculine rights.

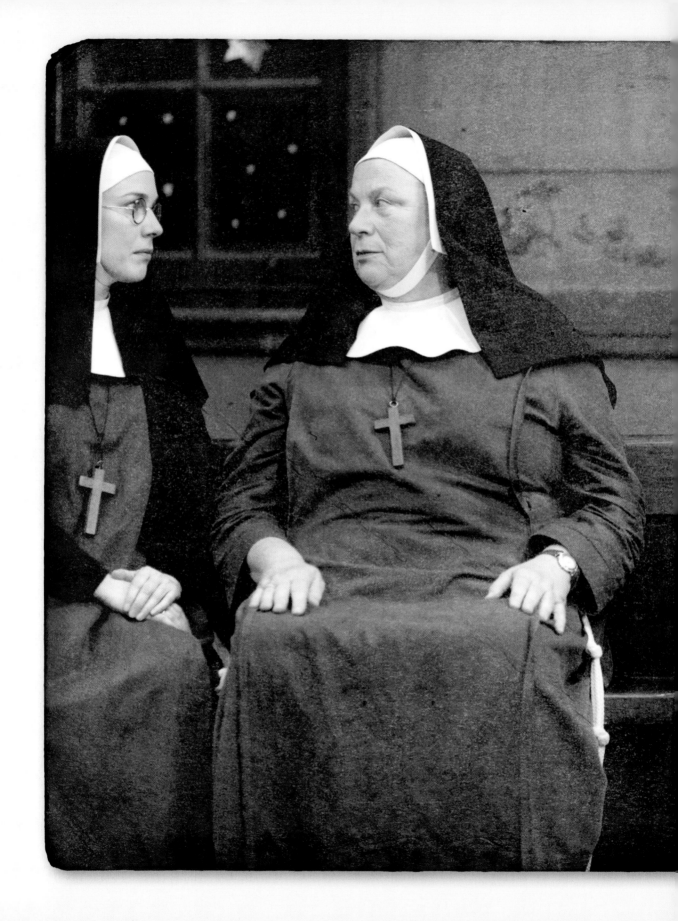

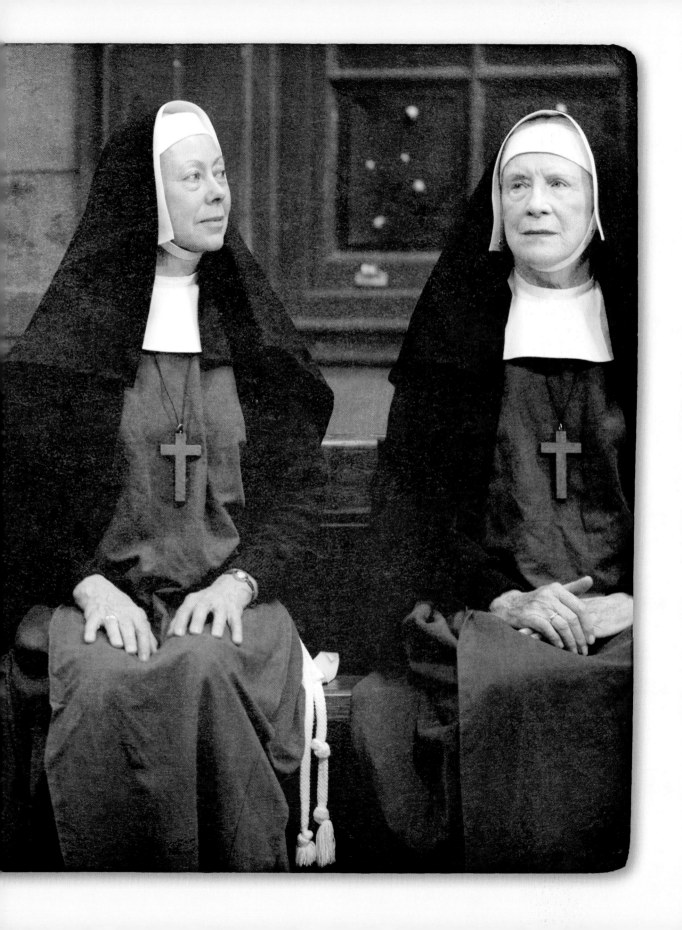

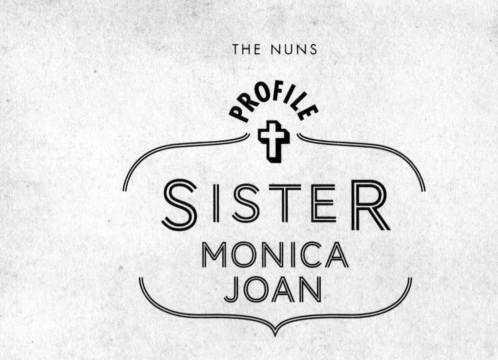

PROFILE ✝ SISTER MONICA JOAN

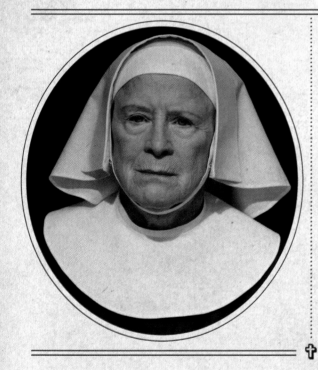

Playing complex, crabby Sister Monica Joan presents an unusual challenge for Judy Parfitt. But with a long pedigree in stage, film and television, she nailed the character at the outset. 'She is mischievous, humorous and highly intelligent. She is very well read and quotes a lot from the classics. She can also be very sharp, in a concealed sort of way.'

Sister Monica Joan's lightning switches from confusion to clarity keep everyone guessing, including Judy. 'She goes in and out of moods and moments. A lot of the time you don't know whether she is naughty and mean, or if she has gone off on her own eccentric path,' says Judy.

Judy has some experience of dealing with dementia as her husband, actor Tony Steedman, suffered from the vascular form before his death in 2001. Yet she has identified differences between the two. 'I know from my husband that, with dementia, you can go off and be a different person and not know you are doing it, and then be rational for a short space of time. But even before dementia Sister Monica Joan sang to her own tune. She is an innocent in many ways, but sometimes very objective and clever.'

Judy's portrayal of Sister Monica Joan is based on deep consideration. 'It isn't a question of learning the lines for this part, it is about going on her journey before you come to work each day. I have to find a truthful way of doing that and it is not something that can be done quickly.'

In a cast where Judy says 'there are no egos' she's made a host of good friends, including comedienne Miranda Hart. During Series One, they got into difficulties by making each other laugh – something actors refer to as 'corpsing'.

'Every time we looked at each other we just giggled. We had to pull ourselves together a bit. It is wonderful fun, until you get to the frightening point that every time you look at each other you laugh. So I thought I would not look into her eyes. But you can't do a scene without looking into her eyes! Eventually we both knew we were holding on by a thread and that makes it even worse.'

Recently Judy has been frequently cast in period dramas – including the Emmy-winning *Little Dorrit*, in which she played cruel Mrs Clennam – and become accustomed to heavy, elaborate costumes. Although she finds her habit very comfortable, there are some disadvantages to convent modes. 'The wimple ruins your hair. I have very curly hair and it is always flattened. And you can't hear anything because you have three different layers over your ears.' She concludes, 'You don't want to look in the mirror a lot.'

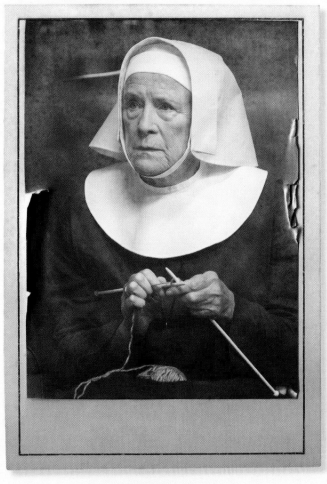

'A lot of the time you don't know whether she is naughty and mean, or if she has gone off on her own eccentric path.'

JUDY PARFITT

Q&A

What are the best things about being a nun?
One finds the quadrants of the spirit so very satisfactorily aligned. And there is also cake.

Is there anything you miss since taking your vows?
I have been in the religious life for more than fifty years. I should be a lamentable specimen if I were still moping and caterwauling over distant trifles.

If you could take a holiday, where would you go?
I should hie myself to Freiberg, to hear the great organ, and from thence to Vienna, to sample the chocolate sponge at the Hotel Sacher. I understand apricot conserve is involved.

Do you have a favourite piece of music or book (apart from the Bible)?
I find John Keats is able to furnish us with a bon mot for most occasions, perhaps the more so because he trained as an apothecary and was baptised at St Botolph's, Bishopsgate.

'No, no! go not to Lethe, neither twist
Wolf's-bane, tight-rooted, for its poisonous wine;
Nor suffer thy pale forehead to be kiss'd
By nightshade, ruby grape of Proserpine ...'
Et cetera.

Do you have time for hobbies?
Hobbies are the final refuge of the idle. I knit, naturally, and have garnered great praise for my gollies. But it is all undertaken for charitable ends.

What's your favourite smell?
The odour of sanctity. Sadly, one seldom encounters it in Poplar.

What's your most treasured memory?
Closing the door on my family home, the day I left to join the Order. I asked our butler to step to one side, and then I slammed it as hard as I could.

What's your secret vice?
If Sister Bernadette mentioned the gramophone record by Mr Perry Como, then I am pained to say that she is telling falsehoods.

And your dearest wish?
To witness the day of Judgement. Revelation promises a most intriguing range of spectacular occurrences, although it vexes me that refreshments are not mentioned.

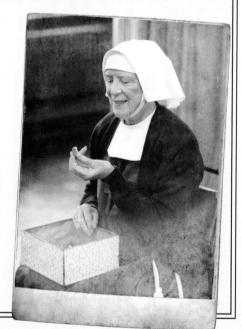

PROFILE
✝
SISTER
BERNADETTE

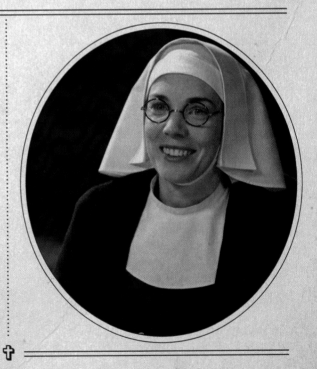

We cast Laura Main as Sister Bernadette on the strength of her acting. Her warm Aberdeenshire accent was an added extra. What we didn't realise was that she had a hidden talent – she can sing.

Laura has considerable experience in musical theatre, making her debut as a child as a Von Trapp in *The Sound of Music*. She recently appeared in the Stephen Sondheim musical *Company*. But neither she nor we knew she was capable of plainsong.

We had originally included scenes of the nuns at prayer in just two episodes. David Ogden, a specialist singing consultant, came to the set to coach the actresses in chanted prayer and the result was so exquisite that I created extra chapel scenes. In all of them, Laura's soprano shines through.

'It was totally unexpected,' says Laura. 'It is so nice to come on TV and get to sing! It took

✝

a while to get the hang of such a different style,' she admits, 'but people that know me recognised my singing voice.'

Laura herself is never recognised in mufti. 'When your costume is glasses and wimple, you don't get recognised.' This is something she enjoys. 'There's a freedom in not being concerned with your appearance. As a woman it is good to do something in which it's your acting, and not your looks, that counts.'

Sister Bernadette is close in age to the young midwives, but will always be on the fringes of their group. 'In the first series there was a scene where Sister Bernadette was looking at all the girls going off to the dance. When she is left alone, she removes her headdress and looks at herself in the mirror. That was the moment that showed you so much more of her than before. It was such an intimate, private moment.'

Laura herself confesses to a quiet faith. At Easter 2012 she took part in a broadcast service at Canterbury Cathedral, called *At the Foot of the Cross*. Her readings included Bible passages from Isaiah and Matthew, and the Anglo-Saxon poem 'The Dream of the Rood'. To her delight, she returned home to find her whole family huddled round the radio, listening in.

Family is very important to Laura. Cradling babies in *Call the Midwife* holds no fears for her – she is an experienced and very hands-on aunt to toddler nephews James and Ross, and new niece Ashleigh, born in February 2012.

'Once I was tentative about holding babies. But when you are an aunt you just have complete rapport with these children.' She smiles, her blue eyes lighting up. 'Oh, I love being an auntie.'

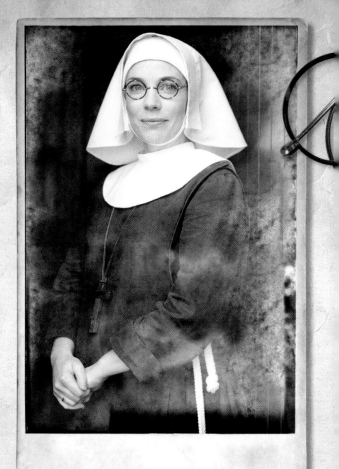

Sister Bernadette is close in age to the young midwives, but will always be on the fringes of their group.

✝

Q&A

What are the best things about being a nun?
The services of prayer we have throughout the day, beginning with Lauds at dawn, and ending with Compline before we go to bed. They provide us with such solace and such inspiration and are a constant reminder of why we do this, and for whom.

Is there anything you've missed since taking your vows?
There are many things I miss, but more that I have found.

If you could take a holiday, where would you go?
Somewhere with palm trees. Torquay would suffice.

Do you have a favourite piece of music or book (apart from the Bible)?
As midwives we often receive little gifts from grateful patients, and not long ago I was given a record of Perry Como singing 'Ave Maria'. We listened to it during recreation and everyone thought it very nice indeed. The next day I came into the parlour and caught Sister Monica Joan dancing to the B-side, which was a rather jaunty song called 'Do You Ever Get That Feeling In The Moonlight?'. So I suppose that's my favourite, because it makes me smile.

Do you have time for hobbies?
I've a nice line in tea cosies, which I make in handicrafts.

What's your favourite smell?
Laundry starch, which is just as well because our wimples are rigid with it. The smell of starch follows me everywhere I go.

What's your most treasured memory?
The sound of my mother's voice calling me to come in when it was getting dark.

What's your secret vice?
I sing in the bath. I have to put a towel against the bottom of the door and keep turning on the taps so nobody can hear me.

And your dearest wish?
To continue in God's grace. Without faith, I can do nothing.

Sister Bernadette

CHAPTER
5
HEALTH

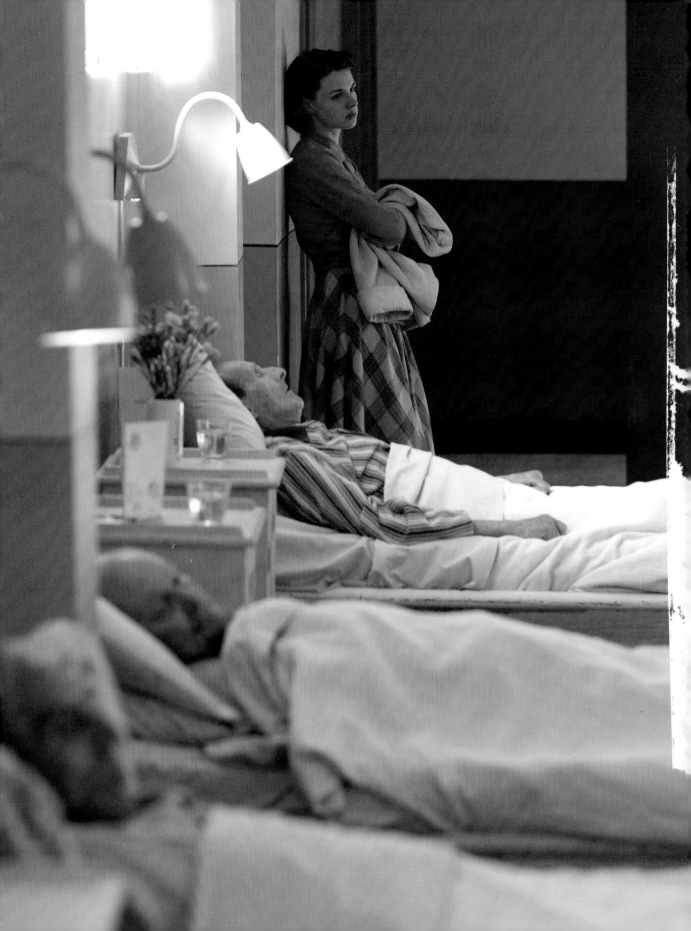

HEALTH

'I WILL NOT HAVE ROTTING
MATTER PUT INTO MY VEINS!'

SISTER MONICA JOAN

'IF YOU WON'T ACCEPT THE PENICILLIN THEN
YOU WILL BE ROTTING MATTER!'

SISTER EVANGELINA

When we started developing the scripts for *Call the Midwife*, we did not consciously intend it to promote the NHS. We were, after all, making a drama set in 1957 – just ten years into this great social experiment. At that point not only was the National Health Service newly up and running in the most spectacular way, but the casualties of the old, unfunded system were still very much in evidence. The dramatic possibilities were obvious, and it was easy to simply portray it from the perspective of the time – the National Health was an absolute good.

Pippa Harris, our Executive Producer, comes from a distinguished medical background; her father, Dr Tony Harris, was a prominent psychiatrist and her grandmother, the Hon. Noel Olivier, one of the first female doctors to qualify in England. Pippa kept a keen eye on the medical content of the show, but, as she observes, 'In the fifties, some aspects of medicine were still quite raw. We thought audiences would be shocked by childbirth without pain relief, and cancer without much hope of cure. To our surprise, the audience were filled with real affection for this very different time.'

After *Call the Midwife* was broadcast, a veritable roar went up – we had clearly touched some sort of common nerve. There was suddenly a great deal of analysis in the papers, comparing past standards of healthcare with those of the present day. Overwhelmingly, it was felt that not all change has been for the better. Comments were not just confined to midwifery, but touched on general nursing, GP care and the Welfare State at large. *Call the Midwife*'s 'Fabian' – that is to say left-wing – stance was also praised in some reviews. Philippa Lowthorpe, our lead director, was overjoyed. 'Quite honestly, I felt like cheering!

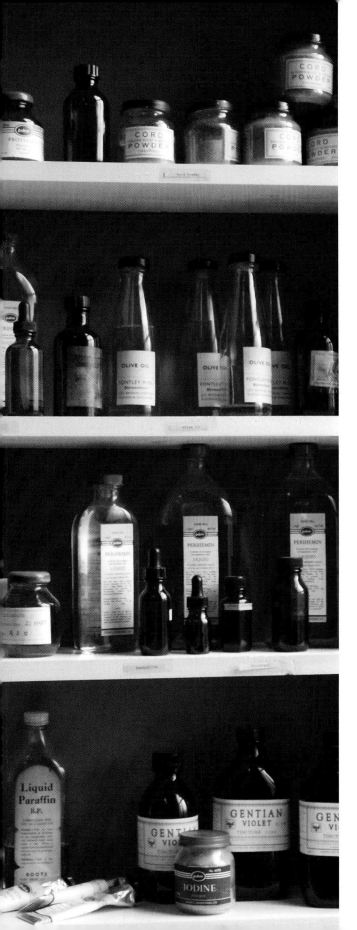

Ordinary working people, like those attended by the nuns and the nurses of Nonnatus House, had every reason to rejoice.

When we are working on this show, we can't forget how precious the NHS is, how many lives it has saved and how many people it has helped.'

The concept of the National Health Service was bold and ambitious. It undertook to provide the best possible medical care for rich and poor alike, free of charge, from the cradle to the grave. Its principles were set down during World War Two, but it took a Labour government to bring it to fruition, and it was finally unveiled in July 1948.

Ordinary working people, like those attended by the nuns and the nurses of Nonnatus House, had every reason to rejoice. Doctors, pharmacists, opticians, dentists and hospitals were now available to them. They were entitled to surgery, hearing aids, dentures, spectacles, walking sticks, wheelchairs. They could have back braces, corsets, vitamins, wigs. If their children had knock-knees, they would get remedial shoes. If they were plagued with catarrh, out would come their adenoids. Things were looking up for everyone, but the lives of the very poorest were utterly transformed.

Health insurance had been introduced nationally in 1911, but the scheme was patchy and many suffered. Free treatment was offered by certain hospitals, and kind-hearted doctors might 'forget' to leave a bill. Nevertheless, there was an enormous gulf between the needs of the people and the state's ability to provide it. This had to be bridged by private endeavour. My own grandfather was a medicinal herbalist, operating out of a shop in Garston, Liverpool until the 1930s. We still have his faded book of remedies, detailing emulsions for skin complaints, linctus for chestiness and potent blends of vinegars for fever. He made a cracking cough mixture, but could he have cured scarlet fever or anaemia? Could he have dealt with gallstones, or with meningitis? The tragedy was not that he probably tried, but that he had to. Those on limited incomes had nowhere else to turn.

In *Call the Midwife*, one of the reasons why the Nonnatuns are so cherished is because they've been in Poplar for over sixty years. In 1957 we see them working hand in hand with the National Health. However, like their real-life counterparts the Order of St John the Divine, they had long been a lifeline for the people of East London.

Women in particular needed every ounce of help on offer. Until the Midwives Act was passed in 1902 – after no fewer than 11 attempts to get it passed in Parliament – midwifery was not a certifiable profession. Anyone with even basic knowledge could set herself up as 'midwife' and collect a fee. Training was not required, techniques were often primitive and hygiene was precarious at best.

The more urban the district, the higher the rate of infant mortality. In densely populated Preston, Lancashire, in 1890, 223 babies in every 1,000 live births would die. Stillbirths were registered only haphazardly, but in that same year, fifty out of every 1,000 labouring mothers did not survive. Much of the damage was done by unscrupulous amateur midwives, nicknamed 'gamps' after Sarah Gamp, the brutal nurse in Dickens's *Martin Chuzzlewit*. Unskilled and unclean, they still claimed a few shillings for their time, no matter how badly they botched the delivery, preying on the poor and vulnerable.

It is entirely fair to say that these were not the only women delivering babies. Until the late 19th century, all women relied on 'wise women' from their community, who had been taught by the previous generation and gathered expertise over the years. Some districts came up with hybrid solutions to the problem. Sister Christine Hoverd, a midwife with the original Order of St John in Poplar, remembered her own grandmother working as a 'handy woman' in the years between the wars.

> *Until the Midwives Act was passed in 1902, midwifery was not a certifiable profession.*

'Midwifery was developing,' Christine Hoverd explains, 'but not all country areas had the joy of a proper midwife. My grandmother would follow the doctor, going into a house when the woman was in labour, and stay for a number of days afterwards. I remember her going out in this big white apron, ready to look after a mother.'

But the fact remains that only some women could stretch to hiring a doctor.

THE EVOLUTION OF HEALTHCARE AND WOMEN'S RIGHTS IN BRITAIN

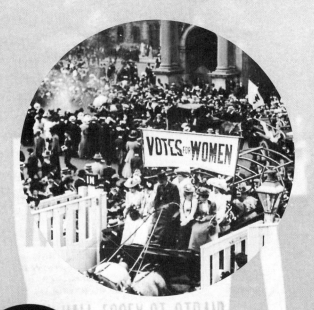

Eleanor Davies-Colley, appointed House Surgeon at the New Hospital for Women in 1907, is the first woman to be admitted to the Royal College of Surgeons.

MIDWIVES ACT

In June 1908, a rally of more than 250,000 gathers in Hyde Park on 'Women's Sunday' to support women getting the vote.

NATIONAL INSURANCE ACT

On 31 July 1902, Parliament passes the Midwives Act, which gives midwifery legal recognition and regulation for the first time.

National Insurance is introduced. Part 1 of the Act gives 15 million low-paid workers the right to free medical treatment, and Part II of the Act gives people the right to receive unemployment benefit. The Act also introduces a thirty-shilling maternity benefit.

1902

1908

1911

WOMEN WIN EQUAL VOTING RIGHTS

WOMEN OVER 30 GET THE RIGHT TO VOTE

At the end of the war, the Representation of the People Act is passed, which gives women over 30 the right to vote. It only represented 40 per cent of the total population of women in the UK.

The Equal Franchise Act is passed, and women are given the same voting rights as men.

FAMILY ALLOWANCE ACT

The Family Allowance Act introduces welfare payments for families.

NATIONAL INSURANCE ACT 1946

The National Insurance Act establishes a comprehensive system of social security in the UK.

1918

1928

1945

1946

CONTINUED >>

THE EVOLUTION OF HEALTHCARE AND WOMEN'S RIGHTS IN BRITAIN

Your NEW Health Service!

POLIO AND DIPHTHERIA VACCINES LAUNCHED

The landmark programme ensures everyone under the age of 15 is vaccinated.

NATIONAL HEALTH SERVICE CREATED

One shilling charges are brought in for prescriptions.

Health Minister Aneurin Bevan officially launches the NHS on 5 July 1948, the first health system to offer publicly funded medical care to the entire population.

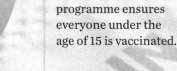

PROTECT YOUR CHILD FROM DEADLY DIPHTHERIA

Have your child immunised against this dreadful scourge which attacks 50,000 children yearly in Great Britain between 2,000 and 3,000 deaths. Imm... protection. It involves mere...

1948

1952

1958

The contraceptive pill is available on prescription from the NHS at a subsidised cost of two shillings a month.

RUBELLA VACCINATION UNVEILED

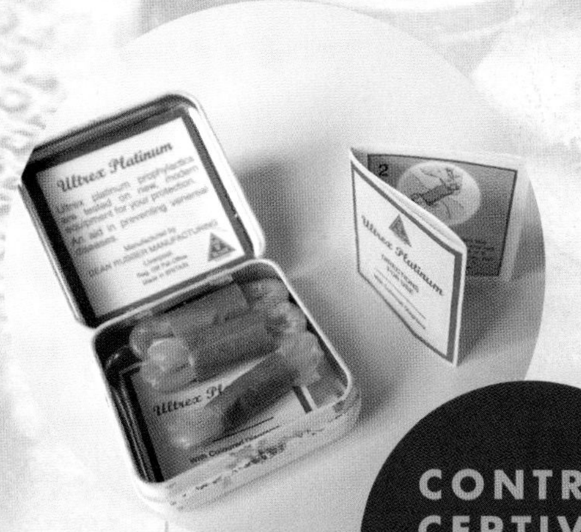

FIRST ORAL VACCINE FOR POLIO

The oral polio vaccine, created by Dr Albert Sabin, is administered on sugar cubes.

First vaccine made available for measles.

First vaccine made available for mumps.

CONTRA-CEPTIVES AVAILABLE ON NHS

1961

1962

1963

1967

1970

1974

Others paid for what they could afford – and took a chance.

Public pressure in Britain started with the Midwives Institute, founded in 1881, which aimed to garner support for training and registration. Ten years later, the number of trained midwives had reached 1,000, but support for them was far from universal. Mrs Bedford Fenwick, a former matron at London's St Bart's Hospital, called midwives 'an anachronism' and 'a historical curiosity'.

'A startling statistic was that in this area of Poplar there were 150 to 200 births every month. After the pill, that dropped to four or five.'

PAM FERRIS
Sister Evangelina

However, abiding concerns about the health of the nation were raised by a powerful lobby, the army. Sickly infants make for sickly adults, and the poor calibre of men presenting for service in the Boer War became perturbing. One-third of army applicants were rejected, so military top brass raised the alarm and, with infinite slowness, the wheels began to turn. By 1957, midwifery training was excellent and highly regulated. Today, a copy of Margaret Myles' seminal *Textbook for Midwives* has pride of place on our set.

The NHS was part of a broad plan conceived by William Beveridge during the War to conquer the domestic 'enemies of the state'. These were identified as want, disease, squalor, ignorance and idleness. Everyone agreed pre-war services were inadequate and poorly coordinated, but there was still opposition to the National Health proposal. It would be funded from taxation, which is never popular, and some GPs feared that their income would suffer, while an increased workload would compromise patient care. Other, more idealistic doctors saw past these immediate hurdles. They looked forward to the widespread prevention and cure of disease, and towards sunny uplands promising health for all.

One enormous leap forward was the increased availability of contraception. In Series One, Chummy tried to persuade the wives of Poplar to embrace the condom. We saw her gamely brandishing a wooden penis and a contraceptive sheath, but her audience were unconvinced. Much as they would like fewer pregnancies, they knew their men weren't keen to compromise their pleasure.

On the first birthday of the NHS, Health Minister Aneurin Bevan conceded that it had been started in 'an atmosphere of friction, controversy, doubt and of great hopes.' At that stage, it still had its teething problems, notably shortages, over-crowded waiting rooms and a lack of surgical facilities. *Call the Midwife*'s 'pop-up' maternity clinic in All Saints Parish Hall – where sessions are squeezed between carpet bowls and dancing classes – is a testament to this. But Bevan robustly defended the creation of the Service.

'Most of the shortcomings which have been revealed by the British Health Service are not the result of the intrinsic defects of the service, but because of the overwhelming volume of need that the service has revealed … There has gone on, in the past, a vast amount of silent suffering.'

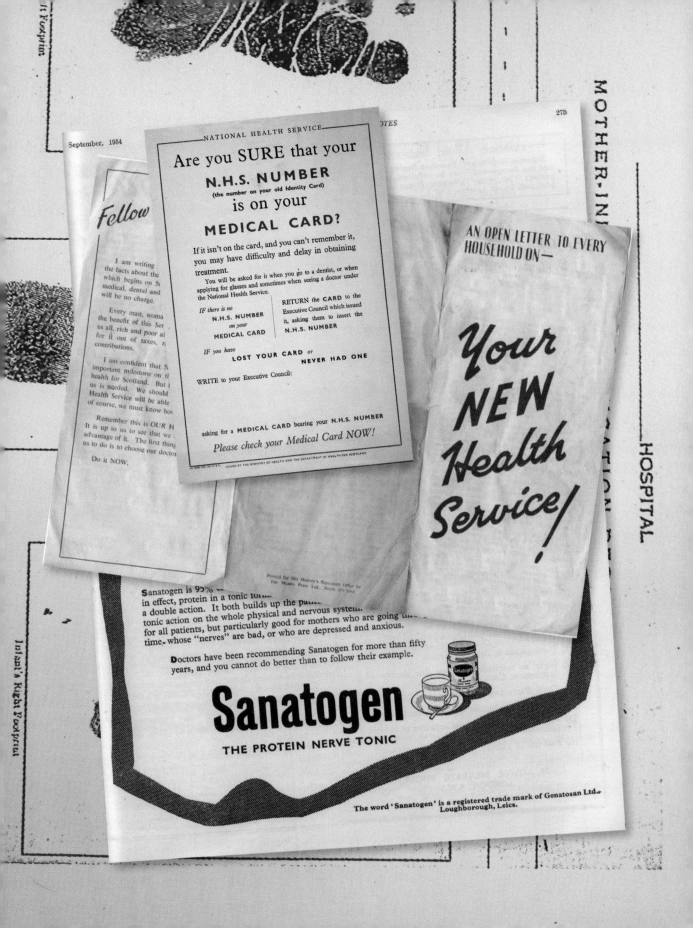

Subjective
warmth and

DRINK EVERY DAY
MILK
for health

AND ALL THE BETTER FOR IT

PENICILLIN SQUIBB
(Sodium Salt of Penicillin
Contains 10,000 Florey units
No Preservative
KEEP BELOW 45°F.
Caution: New Drug—Limited
federal law to investigational use.
E.R. Squibb & Sons, N.Y.
Biological Laboratories,
New Brunswick, N.J.

...nd other manifestations

...yton House, Euston Rd., N.W.1   *Wyeth*

A Royal Year for Immunisation

"Prince Charles, who will be a year old on November 14th, has recently been inoculated against diphtheria."

**EXTRACT FROM "The Times"
OF 21ST OCTOBER, 1949.**

Every baby in the land should be protected before he is a year old. The family doctor or Welfare Centre will advise any mother.

Issued by THE MINISTRY OF HEALTH

"Your Welfare is Our Concern"

For 70 years this has been the guiding principle of

THE ROYAL COLLEGE OF MIDWIVES

(Patron: HER MAJESTY QUEEN ELIZABETH THE QUEEN MOTHER)

RCM
1881
VITA · DONUM · DEI

Membership of the College will bring you many advantages including :

(1) Participation in Branch activities.

(2) Right to nominate and vote for election of Members to Council.

(3) Third Party Indemnity Insurance Cover.

(4) Expert help and advice on professional matters.

(5) Participation in educational activities at reduced fees.

(6) Free use of Library.

**57 LOWER BELGRAVE STREET,
LONDON, S.W.1**
Telephone : SLOane 8313

SUBSCRIPTION :

(i) Headquarters members : 26s. per annum.
(ii) Branch members : 21s. per annum payable to Headquarters plus Branch subscription.
(iii) Overseas members : 5s. per annum.
(iv) Pupil midwives : 2s. 6d. per annum.

FILL IN THIS FORM AND POST TO-DAY

...ME A MEMBER OF THE ROYAL
...GE OF MIDWIVES

Name ....
Address
(BLOCK
CAPS.) ....
Remittance enclosed ....   Headqu...
Branch
Overseas
Pupil Midwife

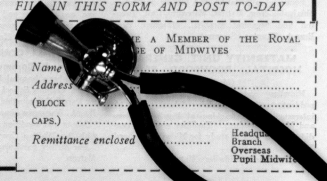

The original *Call the Midwife* books carried several stories that amply illustrated this, and provided some of the most harrowing and moving material for the series. Ancient Mrs Jenkins, half-mad with self-neglect, hobbling on eight-inch toenails. Old soldier Joe Collett, losing his legs because of unhealed army wounds. And gentle Brenda McEntee – her body deformed by rickets – who endured consecutive stillbirths because she couldn't afford a doctor's help.

Brenda's story in Series One was exceptionally moving. We saw her weeping with terror at the clinic – her child had begun to move in her womb, something she experienced with all four of the children she lost at birth. She found it hard to believe that she might be helped. Her grief was still raw and Chummy had to step in with calming words. At the end of the episode, we were shown Brenda's beautiful thriving newborn, born by Caesarean section for which there was no charge. The NHS gave her the gift of motherhood.

Rickets, which is now almost unknown in the developed world, was a common childhood disease of poverty. It led to stunted growth and extensive skeletal deformity caused by a lack of Vitamin D. Vitamin D is principally derived from sunlight, oily fish and dairy produce, all of which were thin on the ground for impoverished children in the inner city. Tragically, girls were more prone to rickets than boys – from a young age they would be kept indoors, looking after the smallest siblings while their brothers played out, running wild and swimming naked in canals. This gave them just enough of the precious vitamin, but their sisters' skeletons – like Brenda's – softened and buckled, deforming them for life and making childbirth fraught.

From the middle of the 20th century, huge strides were made in the prevention of rickets. From 1944, the British government issued free milk to all school children up to the age of 18 years. With the advent of the NHS, free orange juice was made available through public clinics, along with cod liver oil. Wildly unpopular with its recipients, this thick, fishy liquid put the last nail in the coffin of the dreaded rickets. From the very commencement of the NHS, prevention and cure went hand in hand.

In 1958, the NHS had about 22,000 GPs on its books. They cost £72 million a year, one tenth of its entire budget. Each doctor cared for an average of 2,200 patients and was paid £1 per head on surgery lists. In teeming urban districts such as Poplar, they had their work cut out, but they did not toil alone.

Rickets, now almost unknown in the developed world, was a common childhood disease of poverty.

In *Call the Midwife*, harried Dr Turner is at once supported and inspired by the Sisters of Nonnatus House. Their midwifery work goes hand in hand with serving the district on a general medical level. Together with Dr Turner, they make a formidable team. Their success in social medicine is helped by the advent of powerful new drugs.

The most significant of these was penicillin, which was identified by Alexander Fleming in 1928, when he spotted the unexpectedly beneficial effects of mould. There was some early suspicion of the drug, because of its dubious provenance. In Series One, Sister Monica Joan is alarmed when she is prescribed it for pneumonia.

'I will not have rotting matter put into my veins!' she cries.

'If you won't accept the penicillin you will BE rotting matter!' retorts Sister Evangelina, poised to inject it into her petrified thigh.

Sister Monica Joan need not have worried. War has a way of accelerating medicine, and the drug had already been well tested.

In *Call the Midwife*, Dr Turner – who would have served as a medic in World War Two – is seen dishing out penicillin in almost every episode. For doctors accustomed to battling infection on virtually every front, it was an almost holy weapon. Women and children reaped particular benefits. Fatal post-partum fevers that killed so many were no more, and breast abscesses in lactating mothers could be dealt with, promoting optimal nutrition for infants. Penicillin also became the remedy of choice for doctors treating syphilis. The sexually transmitted disease triggered skin sores, rashes and fevers in new babies, and sometimes – as in Pearl Winston's case – the death of the unborn child.

Penicillin was not the only miracle. Hot on its heels came streptomycin, which tackled a different kind of bacteria, and proved effective against tuberculosis (TB). This widespread and often fatal disease was dubbed 'the white plague'.

In Series Two, *Call the Midwife* features the mass X-ray programme that did so much to tackle TB in the general population. Rolled out in parks and other public places, National Health vans provided a mobile chest X-ray service. They proved surprisingly popular, perhaps because free treatment was then provided for those who were diagnosed as having TB.

The discovery of a polio vaccine and its successful delivery to the general population finally brought the disease, which was killing over 5,000 people a year – predominantly youngsters – to heel. Initially, this vaccine was delivered by injection, as featured in the Christmas episode. From 1962, after the oral version was developed, children were given it on a sugar lump. I still remember the antiseptic tang of this and the fact that I was dressed as a reindeer at the time. The juggernaut vaccination programme stopped for no one and for nothing – not even the infants' nativity play. We had been marched off the stage and lined up, still in our costumes, outside the nurse's office. One of the shepherds spat his sugar out – I imagine he was punished, but I don't doubt he got another dose of vaccine.

That would have been in the mid-to-late sixties. In my mind's eye, the memory looks so much like a scene from *Call the Midwife* that it makes me feel quite old. Equally, though, that one image sums up so much that is precious. None of the children have rickets and they are receiving life-giving care – dropped, without much fuss, into an ordinary day. Social medicine. Not always appreciated but, please God, always there.

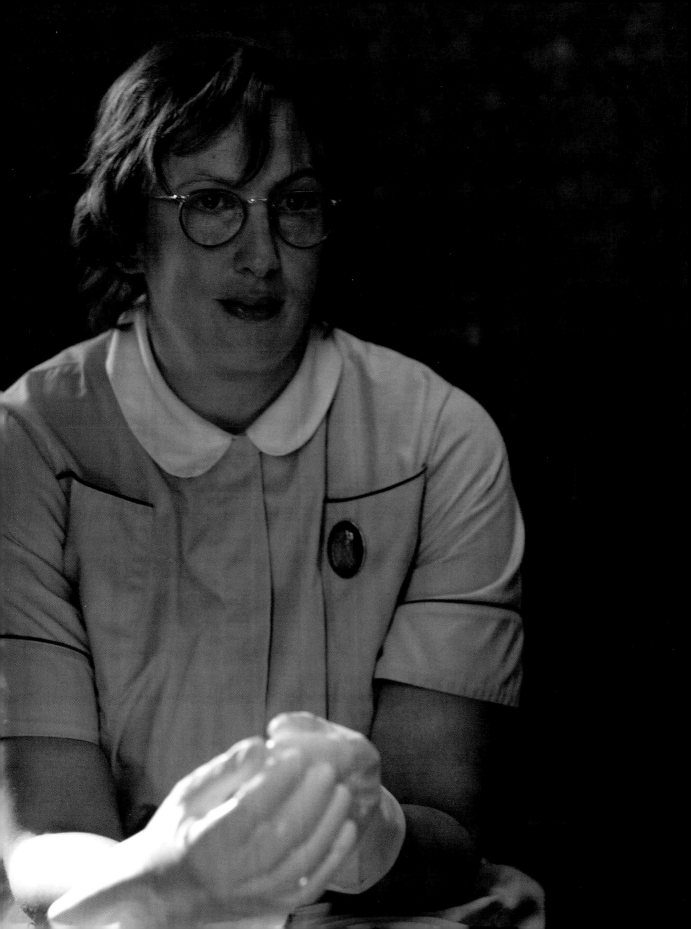

Call the Midwife

Diaries

Part 2

We get a green light at last,
and I am accosted by gypsies.
But our excitement is eclipsed
by tragic news.

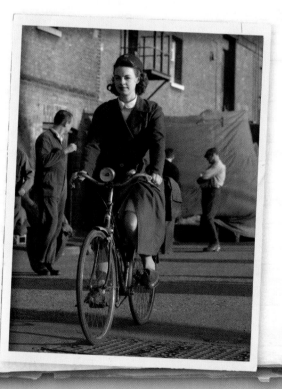

5 December 2009

Pippa says BBC Head of Drama Ben Stephenson has been in touch about *Call the Midwife*. He feels we have a 'problem' with the central character of Jenny Lee. In his view, she is too much of an observer, and not sufficiently interesting in herself.

I broach the subject with Jennifer, who at first totally dismisses the idea of any change. 'The books are not about me,' she says, perfectly horrified. 'They are about the nuns, and the women of the East End! I was just an observer.' We patiently explain that just being an observer doesn't make for very good drama, no matter what you are looking at, and she can see the point of this. As we talk, I realise that one of the most interesting things about Jennifer is that although she is so forthright and even rather frightening these days, she was much more reserved when she was young. I suggest to her that we can work with this in the scripts, showing the young Jenny starting to change and be shaped by her time in Poplar.

Jennifer quite likes this notion. 'It really was the most formative time in my life,' she remarks. Unusually, she goes off on a slight tangent, describing the scene in the East End on Saturday nights. 'Everyone put such an effort into their appearance. The girls would spend all day getting ready, but the Teddy Boys looked rather marvellous too. And, as it went dark, you'd see them all coming out of their houses like fireflies.' Jennifer reveals that she herself went to dances in the crypt of All Saints Church, but enjoyed the dressing up and the preening rather more than the social interaction.

I am left with a haunting image of her standing alone in a room full of noise, working a New Look silhouette. 'I think people thought I was rather standoffish. I suppose it didn't help that I was tall.'

8 December 2009

I make a few careful changes to the script, carving a handful of moments that will flesh out Jenny Lee without betraying the real Jennifer. She approves the amendments — though she is still sad I haven't managed to work in any mention of her navy blue coat with the scarlet lining — and the new draft goes to the BBC.

15 July 2010

More than six months has passed, with no movement on *Call the Midwife*. Ben Stephenson remains both jaunty and supportive, but we seem stuck at a red light, waiting for a green.

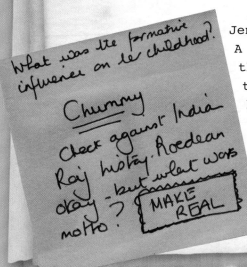

Jennifer doesn't seem remotely daunted. A few weeks ago she called Pippa to say that she had found the perfect actress to play Chummy — a part we always told her might prove difficult to cast. 'I just saw her in a situation comedy' said Jennifer, who never watched much telly. 'I doubt you'll have heard of her, but her name's Miranda Hart, she's six foot two and she falls over splendidly. I think she'd be quite marvellous.' Pippa had to explain to Jennifer that Miranda is in fact a massive star, and probably inundated with such offers. Jennifer told Pippa not to be 'so feeble', and they sent the books and script to Miranda via her agent.

Miranda's agent has e-mailed today to say she loves the character and would like to meet. Our pleasure in this is dimmed by the fact that we don't want to waste her time. Any meeting must wait until filming is a certainty.

11 November 2010

Still nothing about *Call the Midwife*, despite the arrival of a new Controller of BBC One, Danny Cohen. Ben Stephenson and Pippa are convinced that he will like the show, but there is no sign yet of any progress. I strive to be philosophical — after all, *Cranford* took five years to come good. I also remind myself that earlier this year, the same channel greenlit the reincarnation of *Upstairs Downstairs*, which had been a passion project for my friend Piers Wenger and me for quite some time. Operating out of the BBC Studios in Cardiff, we have been working flat out to get a three-hour mini-series filmed and ready for broadcast this Christmas. *Upstairs Downstairs* is the most challenging type of programme to make — period, heavyweight and for a primetime slot

— and there is also a monkey, at the behest of Dame Eileen Atkins.

Jennifer's calls checking up on *Call the Midwife* have slowed to a trickle, and then stopped. I feel bad about this, but when I pluck up courage to telephone and give her the news that there is no news, she crisply remarks that it's actually rather convenient. 'I've been writing another book. It's all about death, so I've had quite enough to keep me occupied.'

I assume she means it — Jennifer is nothing if not truthful — but there's something in her tone that suggests we've led her on a goose chase. I slink back to Cardiff, and the traumas of Eaton Place. I have a bit of a lump in my throat about *Call the Midwife* now. I think it might be time to start letting go.

21 December 2010

Upstairs Downstairs has ended, rather typically, with high drama. Britain is in the grip of blizzards, and Wales has had it worse than most. Today, the Cardiff team must load the master tapes of the completed mini-series onto a van, and dispatch it to London in time for it to arrive by 5pm. If we fail, it won't be ready to be shown at Christmas. The snow is so bad that the team struggle to get into the edit suite, and it is three minutes past one before I get the call to say the van has left, and our job is done. I just sit for a bit, feeling at once both bereaved and relieved; Eaton Place is no longer my concern.

At half past one, the telephone rings. I can't quite believe it: Pippa is telling me *Call the Midwife* is greenlit. The BBC wants six episodes, scheduled for broadcast in January 2012.

17 February 2011

We have our first proper script conference for *Call the Midwife*. Jennifer doesn't feel the need to attend — I have written Episode Two now, and she loves it.

To my pleasure and surprise, the BBC have also commissioned a six-part series of *Upstairs Downstairs*. It is, however, not going to be easy. Eve Stewart and Amy Roberts, who respectively designed and costumed 'Updown', have already signed up for *Call the Midwife*. And the first thing Dame Eileen said when she was told was, 'This time I want a lot more with the monkey.'

Outside Neal Street Productions' offices, I am accosted by gypsies. They press lucky white heather on me, in spite of me saying I lack the means with which to pay. But they won't take it back, and one gypsy grabs my hand. I pull away, ringing on the office buzzer. 'Whatever you do in there, it's going to change your life,' she says. I obviously don't look sufficiently impressed, because she shouts after me. 'Look out for the fifteenth of the month!'

In the office, Pippa introduces me to Hugh Warren, our producer, for the first time. We laugh at the heather, and put it on the shelf, with all of Neal Street Productions' trophies.

7 March 2011

Today, Pippa, Hugh, Tara Cook and the design team gather outside Aldgate Tube. We are driving round what remains of Poplar, seeking potential locations and taking photographs of anything of note. Because of the massive slum clearance in the 1960s, we are working on the assumption that most of the places mentioned in the book will have to be rebuilt elsewhere. Jennifer has been incredibly excited about this as her memories of the docks and the back streets are still vivid, and she is longing to see the world of her youth re-imagined for the screen.

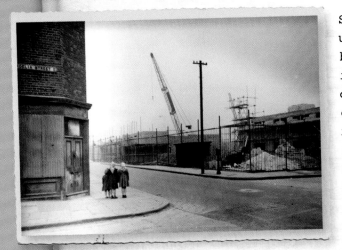

She was supposed to accompany us today, partly as a guide but also because her interest in the show is so immense we couldn't bear to leave her out. However, last night we received an e-mail from Philip saying that Jennifer has been suffering from terrible backache and won't be able to sit in the car. He mentioned that she also has an upset tummy, and says he's going to take her to the doctor. I wonder vaguely if she did herself a mischief last week on her vigorous cycling holiday in Tuscany.

The team have a fascinating day piecing together the remnants of Poplar. We are in high spirits, but I miss Jennifer, the way one misses a friend who's poorly on the day of the school trip.

24 March 2011

In the middle of a flurry of e-mails about *Call the Midwife* and *Upstairs Downstairs* (one of which is headed 'What Are We Going To Do About That Bl**dy Monkey?'), I see something that makes my heart stop. It is a simple subject heading: 'Jennifer: Sad News'. The e-mail is from Pippa. I feel sick even as I open it — we have heard nothing from Jennifer or Philip since she pulled out of the Poplar jaunt. Jennifer has just telephoned Pippa to announce that she has been diagnosed with cancer of the oesophagus, which has already spread to her bones. It is terminal and she has chosen to return home, to be cared for by her family, receiving only palliative care. Pippa asked if it would be all right to tell me, to which Jennifer replied with characteristic crispness, 'Absolutely. There is no point in being secretive about these things.' Pippa said that Jennifer went on to add, without any evidence of sentiment, that she had been looking forward to seeing the finished show enormously, but now thought it unlikely that she would.

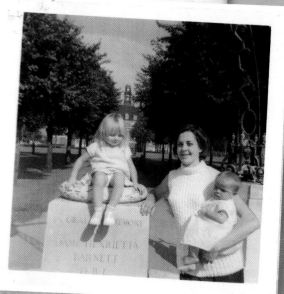

Jennifer Worth and her two daughters, Suzannah (left) and Juliette (right), in 1966.

I look at the completed scripts for Episodes One and Two — the first with all the crossed-out notes in Jennifer's spidery hand, then the second, with practically none. And I can't decipher a single word, for I am blind with tears.

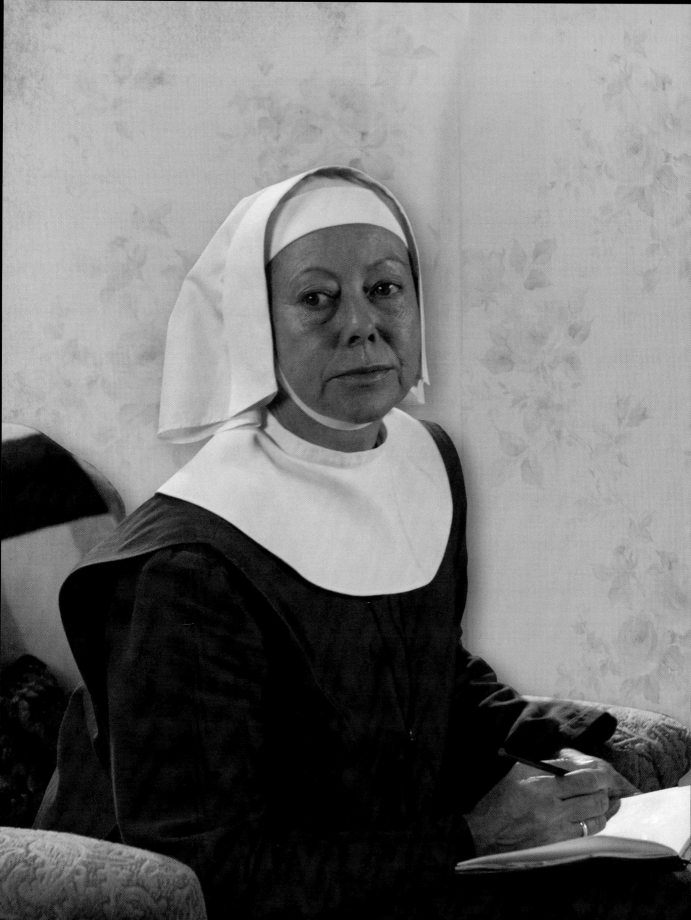

CHAPTER

6

HOMES

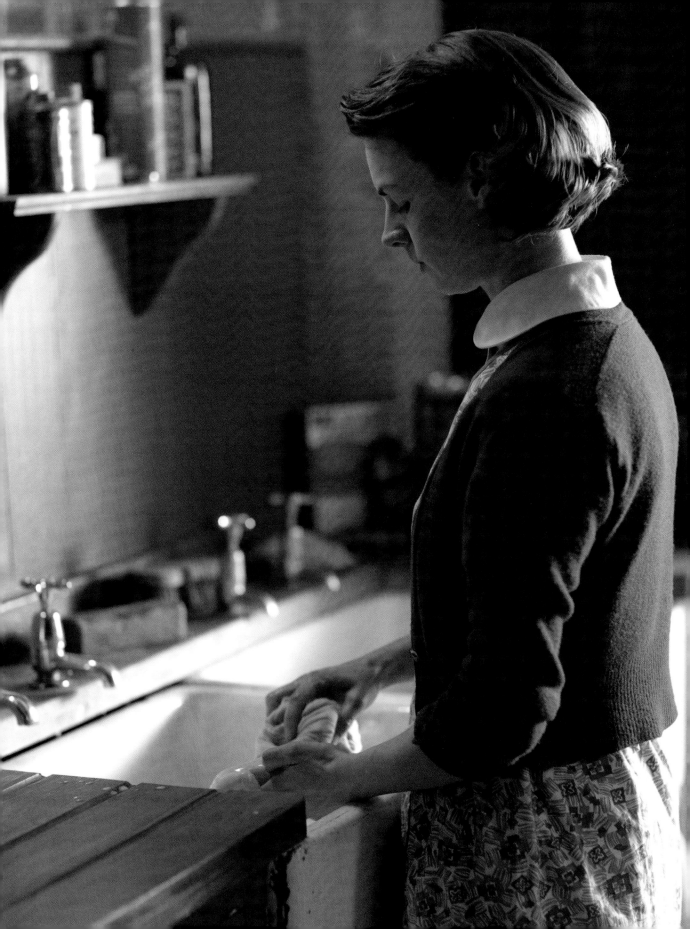

HOMES

'BATHROOM? YOU WERE LUCKY!'
TRIXIE

In terms of set design and props, we perhaps assume the fifties can be evoked with ease. We all know about Ewbanks and bark cloth curtains. We can picture taper-legged tables and plaited plastic mats.

But that is precisely where the challenge lies. As Hugh Warren, producer of *Call the Midwife*, observes, 'It's more difficult to make a show set relatively recently than one set long ago. This is partly because houses were far more cluttered in the 20th century – which means we need to source more props – but also because a lot of the audience have vivid memories of the era.'

Eve Stewart, our production designer, was Oscar nominated for her peerless work on *The King's Speech*, and was the perfect choice for *Call the Midwife*. I was delighted when I heard that our executive producer, Pippa Harris, had invited her on board. 'Great design is vital for a period drama,' explains Pippa. 'You need to convince the audience of the authenticity of what they're watching; to turn a collection of room sets and carefully chosen buildings and streets into an entire cohesive world. Eve is renowned in the industry for her flair, imagination and astonishing attention to detail, and on top of that, she already knew and loved the books, having been brought up in the East End. We couldn't believe our luck!'

Eve makes it her business to capture the way we used to live – from the textures of walls to the art that hangs on them; from the cushions on a chair to the contents of a knitting bag. Her genius is more than just making sure we see a cabbage on the draining board and not new-fangled broccoli. It's more, even, than kitting out a hard-up character with Woodbine cigarettes and not the smarter brand, Park Drive. Eve's attention to

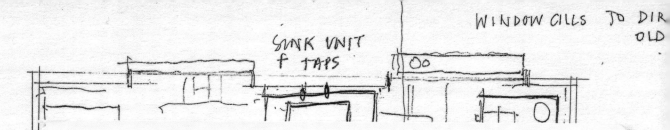

detail is not just relentless, it's celebratory, and this enhances every aspect of the show.

Like everyone involved on *Call the Midwife*, Eve draws on archive photographs, magazines and film for inspiration. But her own background, too, has proved invaluable. Eve's grandmother was in service in London, and her great uncle cleaned windows in the City. Family stories have filtered down through the generations, and her most creative and critical assistants are members of her family. 'I do talk to older relatives – and they are the ones who pick me up the most!'

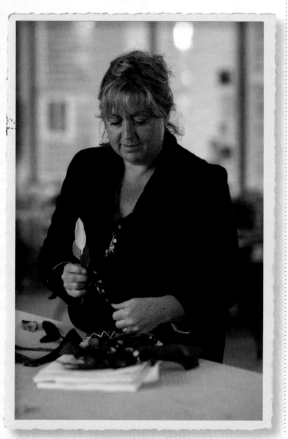

However, Eve always remains creative, led, but not tied down, by facts. 'You have to remember that this is a story; it is a drama first and foremost, not a documentary. We are making a world we want people to believe in, but we have to serve the stories. We try to reflect characters in colours, shapes and textures.'

Under her tireless supervision, Eve's team ensure that postcards adorning East End mantelpieces come from Margate, not Marbella; driving licences are printed on cards, not paper slips. Calendars are created specially, but Eve's team are careful to print them in muted hues – ink was limited in colour in the fifties. Compacts, pencils, buttons and loose change litter sideboards, and there's usually a hairbrush on each mantelpiece.

Eve's attention to detail is not just relentless, it's celebratory. It enhances every aspect of the show.

Eve believes that if a mistake were ever made, the error would be picked up immediately. 'People see so many films and videos today. They may not be able to articulate what is wrong within a certain scene, but they will know something is awry.'

This quiet, relentless work is much respected by the actors. 'The props and design department are extraordinary,' says Jenny Agutter. 'On set one day, in the parlour at Nonnatus House, Pam Ferris and I were talking about things our characters would do. Pam said that Sister

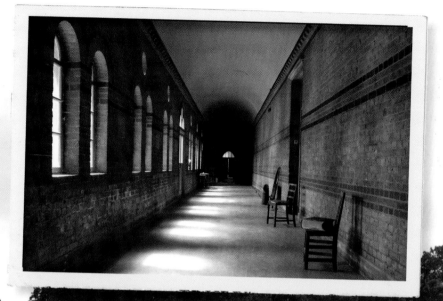

Evangelina would probably collect stamps, whereupon we found books of Green Shield stamps already there on one of the tables. Perfect! It's lovely because it brings the whole thing alive.'

Nonnatus House, and most of *Call the Midwife*'s temporary and standing room-sets, are built at a disused seminary in Mill Hill, North London, which was discovered by our wonderful location manager, Antonia Grant. St Joseph's was opened in the 1870s by a missionary society composed of Jesuits and Redemptorists. From these imposing buildings young men were dispatched across the globe.

Across an undulating meadow, at nearby Holcombe House, they were supported by Franciscan nuns. But during the 20th century the need for missionaries went into decline. In 2006, both convent and seminary were closed. The Jesuit graveyard between the two sites is

a poignant reminder of the past. It is marked with a stark, imposing crucifix, now the perch of choice for London's parakeets and squirrels. As soon as they saw the complex, Eve and Hugh were captivated by its possibilities. Rented together, Holcombe House and St Joseph's now act as location, studio, and technical HQ for *Call the Midwife*.

Whatever production she is working on, Eve, her art director Leon McCarthy and their team of artists move into the studio six weeks ahead of everybody else. Preparations are detailed, painstaking and time consuming. Because the Nonnatus House team are concerned with home delivery, every episode of *Call the Midwife* requires new domestic interiors. For the delivery of Shirley Redmond's daughter Gillian, who was later snatched from her pram, four completely new room sets were required. The sitting room,

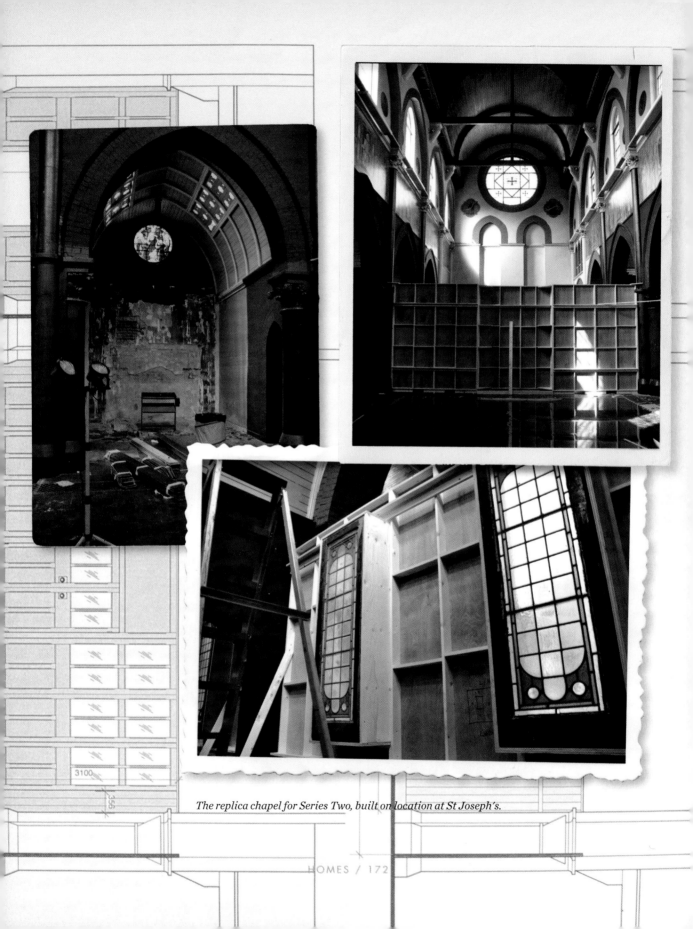

The replica chapel for Series Two, built on location at St Joseph's.

kitchen, hall and bedroom were built by a team of carpenters in otherwise unused chambers at St Joseph's. Though solidly supported, several of the walls were moveable, in order to accommodate cameras and lights.

The tiled Gothic corridors of St Joseph's, with their distinctive high windows, translate straight to the screen as the passageways of Nonnatus House, and in some rooms – such as the area around the telephone desk – the peeling ceiling paper feels just right. Other areas need a lot more work. The chapel in which we see the nuns chant their prayers is pretty, but minute. Filming in it proved so limiting and difficult that a larger replica was built for use in Series Two. All Saints Parish Hall, where the weekly antenatal clinic takes place, is seen in every episode. A former assembly room for missionary students, this is an enormously valuable resource for the show. Eve chose to paint it in a deep muted salmon pink, and then – bearing in mind the wear and tear such a building would receive – gave everything a thorough 'breaking down', scuffing skirtings, adding the odd daub of naughty crayon and painting a large, blackened damp stain by the exit door.

Eve's use of colour is vibrant and distinctive, balancing period veracity with the dictates of television. In the fifties, domestic woodwork was painted in earth tones, rather than brilliant white. During the War, huge quantities of green, grey and brown paint were manufactured for camouflage purposes and for use in military bases – and these were later used up, rather than ditched. In Series One, devoted siblings Frank and Peggy live in a 'prefab', a cheaply made bungalow designed as post-war crisis housing. These flat-pack homes proved both durable and popular, and we filmed their scenes at a surviving prefab in an Amersham museum. The colour

scheme is spot on for the period – dark cream walls and institutional green woodwork.

However, if muddy shades were allowed to dominate on screen, the emotional tenor of the series – which is essentially tender and uplifting – would be undermined. Eve supports the drama by adding luscious slabs of colour to the picture. Nonnatus House has a dark red door, there are bright turquoise walls in the clinical room and Jenny Lee's bed has a grass green counterpane.

While there are very clear rules in place, Eve jumps at the chance to personalise the domestic interiors.

Small details such as towels and bedding – supervised by stand-by art director Bev Gerard – can do much to add a pop of colour to a scene. The art department keep huge quantities of linen in supply, much of it picked up cheaply in markets or on eBay and original to the period. Small details tell big stories – in Series One the striped winceyette sheets on prostitute Mary's bed in the women's refuge were in telling contrast to the stained satin spread in the brothel where we met her.

Wallpaper also needs to be thought through carefully. In Poplar in the fifties, only newlyweds with savings to plunder would have bought the atomic-inspired patterns that were all the rage. In the first series, a design of this type was seen on the curtains in Ingrid Mason's bedroom, when she gave birth to baby Dawn in

Episode Two. 'People in the East End would not have had any spare money. A woman might have been widowed in the First World War and may have redecorated in the early twenties. A couple of years later the Depression started, and that was followed by the Second World War,' Eve points out. 'So people didn't really decorate their houses for a thirty- to forty-year period. By then wallpaper would be marked and peeling.'

While there are very clear rules in place, Eve jumps at the chance to personalise the domestic interiors. In Series One, Len Warren – who fathered 25 children with his Spanish

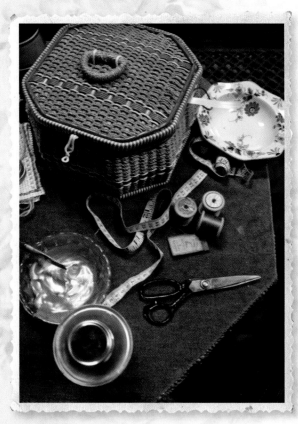

wife Conchita – was a painter and decorator by trade. Although the downstairs reflected the rough and tumble life of an enormous family, it was felt that the upstairs should be a haven for the harried parents. There was a sexual and romantic undertow to their union, and Len had the skills and materials to make the bedroom special. Eve chose a soft primrose yellow for the walls – there would have been little money for rolls and rolls of wallpaper, even at trade prices – but then came up with a delightful defining touch. A pretty floral border was pasted around the room in vertical strips, running from floor to ceiling and dividing the walls into panels. This, to me, said so much about Len and Conchita's relationship – as did the modern vinyl headboard, chosen to highlight the importance of the bed.

Eve always hopes that her own attention to detail will help to sustain the creativity of others. 'We have to make a bubble of belief for the actors. If you get the preparation wrong, if the actors can't believe they are in a house in the East End in the fifties, I don't think they would be that convincing.'

Director Philippa Lowthorpe, who has a background in documentary film making, loves this approach. She also appreciates that in spite of the care that goes into the sets, the stories themselves are never overwhelmed. 'This series is absolutely about people and their lives. They are the most important thing, and they have to stand out.'

Philippa also stresses how the storytelling is helped by skilful lighting, designed by Director of Photography, Chris Seager. 'Chris looks at a scene in an emotional as well as a visual way, relating to the characters and the experience they are having at that point,' she explains.

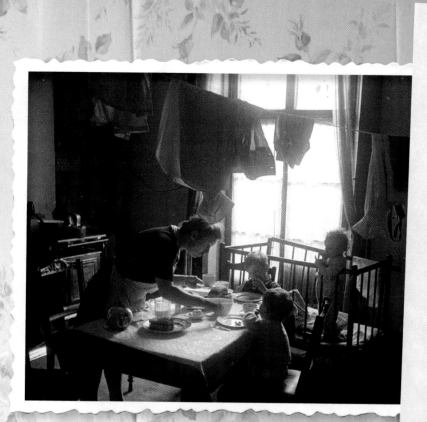

'KNEE PADS.
I SPEND SO MUCH
TIME KNEELING
ON THE FLOOR
DELIVERING BABIES
THEY'VE HAD TO
PROVIDE ME WITH
A SET.'

Jessica Raine

JENNY LEE

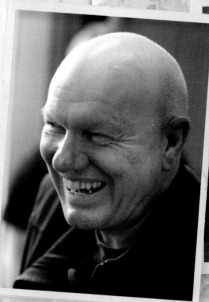

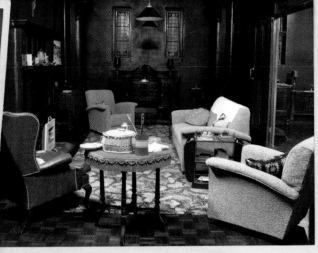

*Above: Chris Seager, Director of
Photography, Series 1 and 2.*

*Overleaf: Sean Baker and Elizabeth Rider,
who played Frank and Peggy in Episode Five.*

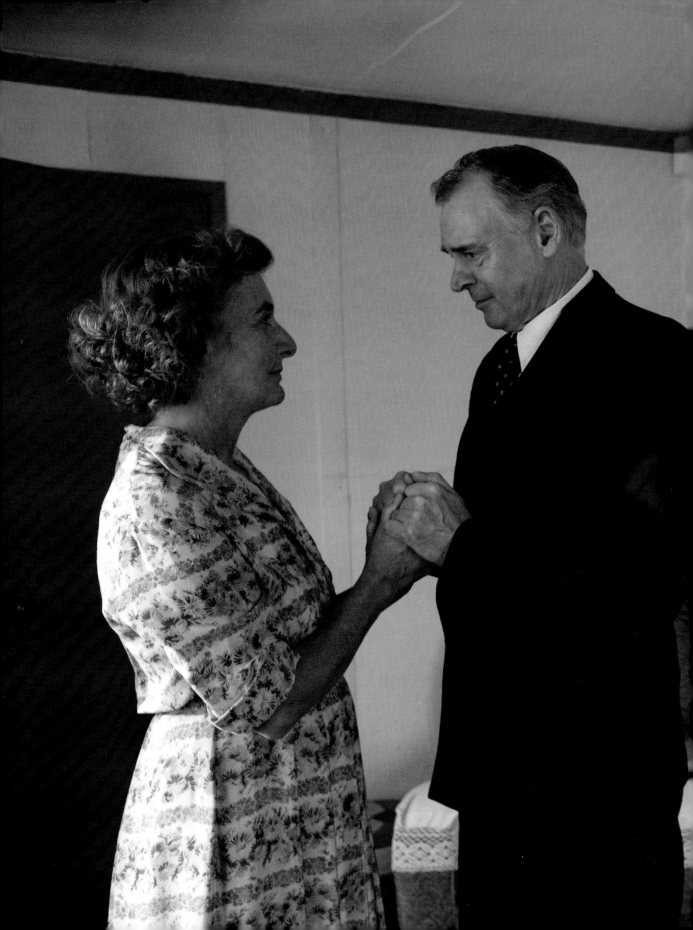

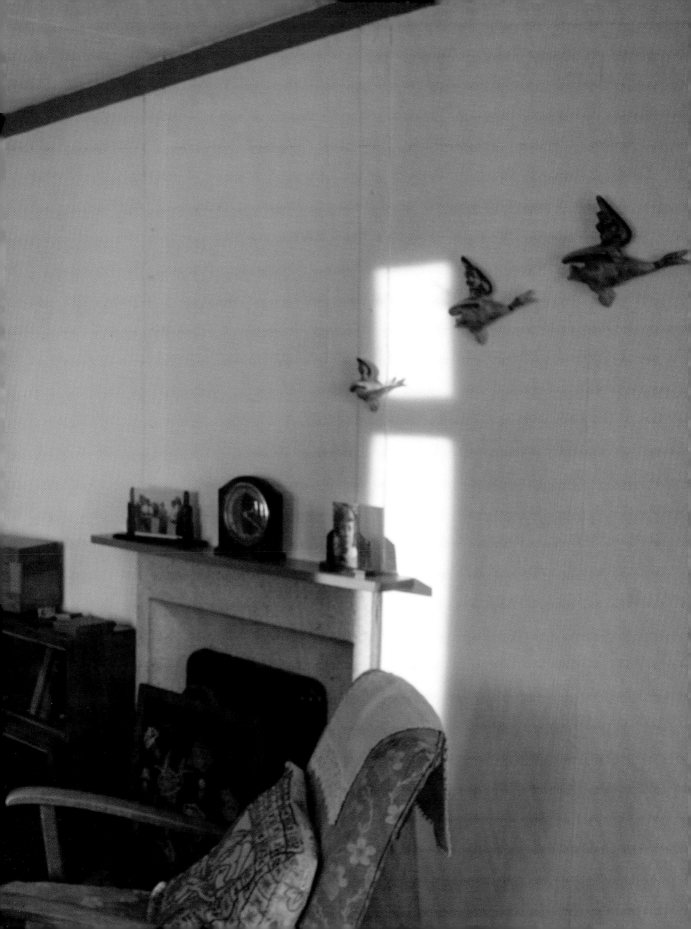

When necessary, the script team go through the characters and their back-stories with Eve before filming begins. Jenny Lee had a secret admirer in Series One – he was never to be seen on screen. However, in the final episode we needed to evoke him simply by showing the contents of his desk. We felt that he had children and this was reflected in the photographs included. He was also an intellectual and a smoker – a blotter and an ashtray were duly supplied. The items were carefully chosen by Eve to indicate that 'Gerald' was several years older than Jenny. Teasing out the little details of the thwarted love affair together, we even gave Gerald an imaginary address, a style of handwriting and chose the ribbon in which Jenny bound his cherished letters. What might have been a mere collection of props became a living, breathing component of the story.

When dealing with larger household objects, such as sofas and kitchen units, Eve may hire

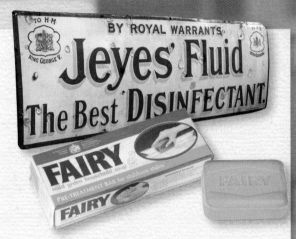

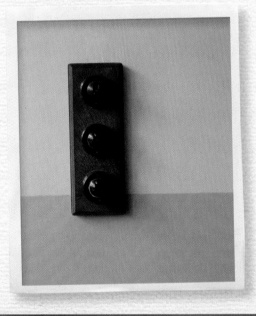

from specialist companies. However, the longer a series runs, the more likely it is that items will be purchased for the sake of continuity. At the outset, prams – like bikes – were tracked down piecemeal and stored in a stairwell at St Joseph's. Our entire collection made a bravura appearance outside the church at Chummy's wedding, when the women of the East End turned out to wish their favourite midwife well. For the second series, a large quantity of vintage prams was bought from a Norfolk-based collector. Neal Street have also invested in ten vintage bikes, to be kept on site and maintained by the crew.

EBay, along with other internet auction sites, is a much valued resource. It has yielded Bakelite light switches, fingerplates and door knobs, all now impossible to purchase off the shelf.

The entire team is perpetually on the hunt for vintage cleaning products, toiletries and other household goods. By the fifties, the days of scrubbing with bicarbonate of soda and vinegar were long gone. Shelves above, or under, every sink were crammed with proprietary potions. Soapless detergent Stardrops had been launched in 1946, though some people still clung to their trusty bars of dark green Fairy. Meanwhile, for those who favoured abrasive methods, there was

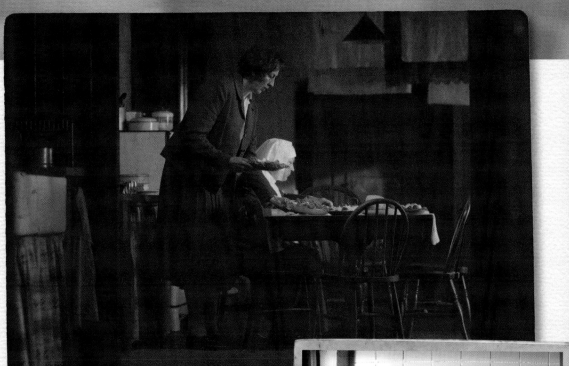

a choice of scouring powders – Vim or Ajax.
A permanent war was waged against bacteria,
with Domestos boasting 'kills all known germs
within the hour', and Jeyes' Fluid claiming to be
'the best disinfectant on earth!'

When dressing the set, if packaging is too
pristine, it must be broken down – a box of
Tide should bear the imprint of wet hands.
Conversely, badly damaged labels can be
reproduced by our inhouse graphic artists.
No branded products are allowed on screen
until they have been through a complex legal
process, and thereby cleared for use.

Overall, kitchens are the most expensive
and difficult domestic interiors to get right,
although this makes the task all the more
rewarding. Prop master Gary Watson managed
to retrieve a five-ring New World gas oven from
Nottingham just in time for Series Two. Eve was

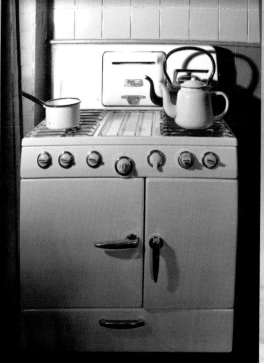

keen that we show Nonnatus House beginning to move with the times, even though the oven no longer works. In the same kitchen the elderly wiring on a fifties' toaster meant it actually posed a hazard. It was therefore manually adjusted, and can now pop out a slice of bread without the need to be connected to the supply. The electric kettle couldn't be plugged in either – instead, a hidden wallpaper steamer produced billowing clouds.

Outside of Nonnatus House, Eve is careful not to include too many labour-saving devices, much as the housewives of Poplar would have loved them. 'People didn't really have much cash. This part of London was slow to catch up, and the economic way of life from some decades earlier persisted.'

The first fully automatic front loader was patented in the States by Bendix. Although manufacture was disrupted by the War, by the

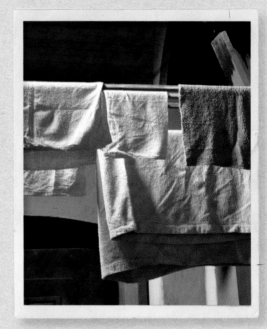

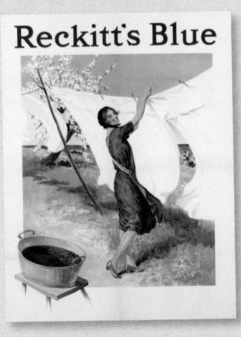

fifties American housewives were breezing their way through their laundry, while their British cousins still wrestled with hand washing. Twin tub washers, which connected to the kitchen taps and left the floor awash, did gain ground in Britain, but at a cost of fifty guineas were a dream for most in Poplar.

'Whites' were a particular source of pride. Women who cared about appearances – and they were legion – would boil sheets, shirts and underwear in a large pot or 'copper', adding a pinch of Reckitt's Blue. This acted as an optical brightener and in skilled hands the effect could be quite dazzling. Stubborn stains were tackled with a brisk rub against a ribbed glass washboard, a process rather hazardous to buttons. In Series One, to Jenny's dismay, Conchita Warren used her pans for boiling laundry in the mornings and cooking stew at night.

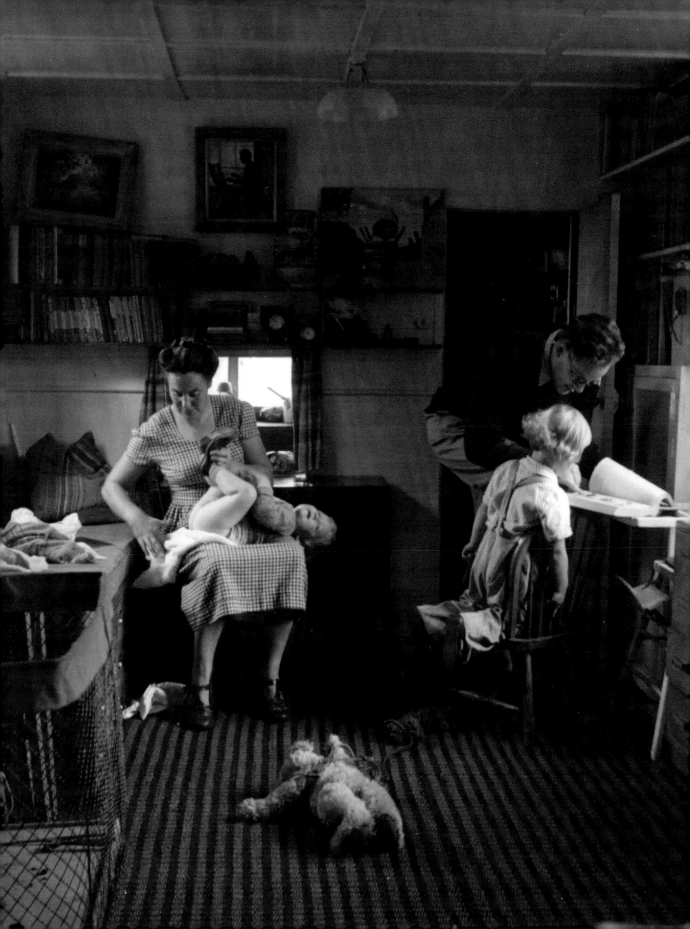

Nappies were a particular trial, especially in homes without a bathroom or scullery. They had to be soaked in a series of lidded buckets, then boiled on the stove, mangled to squeeze out excess water, and dried on a washing line, or indoors by the fire. As a result, babies were toilet-trained early, often being 'out of nappies' by the age of 15 months. And like unlucky Pearl Winston in Series One, some mothers gave up the fight and let toddlers roam with nothing on their bottom half at all.

Even when the washing was dry, the struggle wasn't over. Electric irons were becoming common in the fifties but were costly. Some women still used heavy, rough flat irons heated on the hearth. These veered between scorching fabric at the lightest touch and making no impact on creases at all. Aluminium slip-on covers, which went some way towards updating the device, appeared in the War and remained in service.

Eve and her team are more likely to add a few cobwebs and some dust than to sweep them away, but fifties housewives had other ideas. Polish that usual contained beeswax came in tins and jars, rather than spray form, and brands such as Ronuk and Mansion led the way. Vacuum cleaners like the globe-shaped Hoover Constellation promised more than they delivered, but were finding a place in British homes.

Since the 1920s, if a family owned a gramophone, it would be highly prized and kept in the parlour for best. In the fifties, a new generation of portable Dansette record players came on to the market and became objects of intense desire for teenagers.

Records were measured by rotations per minute on the turntable. Cumbersome 78 rpm records, made with brittle shellac, were the preserve of old-style recording artists. Dropped on a tiled floor, these were inclined to shatter. In the fifties they were superseded by lightweight vinyl that did not crack, but was easy to scratch. 'Singles' were played at 45 rpm, and the new long-playing records at 33 rpm. Well into the 1980s, players were manufactured that could play discs at all three speeds. Artists like Elvis Presley, Pat Boone and Chuck Berry were popular among the young.

While editing Series One, the team became increasingly fond of close-harmony American vocal groups such as the Four Aces and the Five Satins. This transporting and optimistic music with its lush strings, romance and whiff of glamour seems to capture the essence of the fifties.

> *In the fifties, portable Dansette record players became objects of intense desire for teenagers.*

The *Call the Midwife* credits now roll to songs such as 'Stranger In Paradise' – played over Conchita and her thriving baby – and 'Love Is A Many Splendoured Thing', picked for Chummy's triumphant cycle ride. We choose these last of all, often in the cutting room, with the help of editor David Thrasher. For the producers, there is always a sense at this point of a task completed and a job well done. But for Eve, the next phase is already under way. The pressure on her department is perpetual.

'We work 12 hours a day,' says Eve. 'But we have to keep on going. We are like pit ponies, we keep going in the dark.' Then with a very un-fifties' twinkle she adds, 'It's like having a supertanker up your backside.'

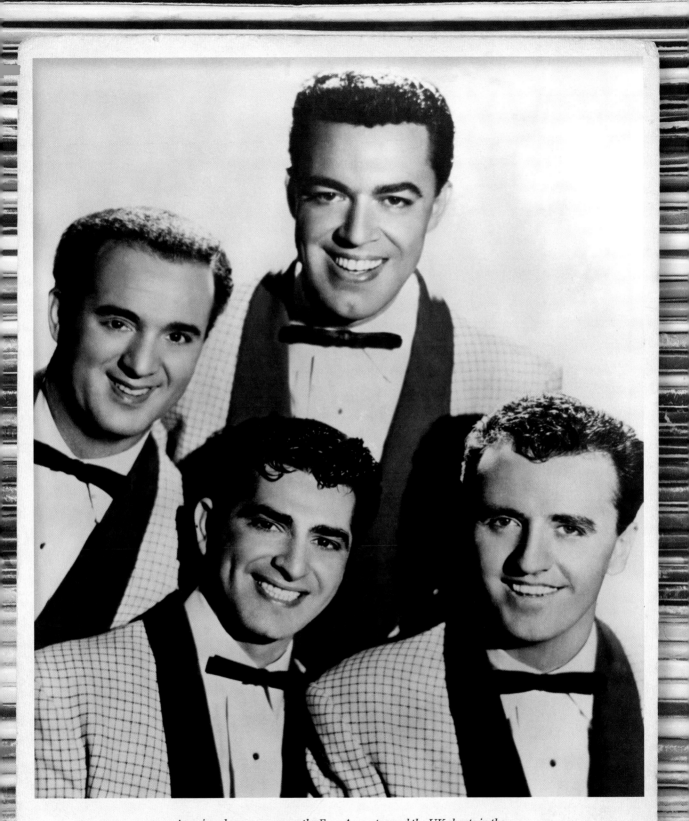

American harmony group, the Four Aces, stormed the UK charts in the mid-1950s. Their biggest hit was 'Love is a Many Splendoured Thing'.

THE SOUNDTRACK

Peter Salem composed the theme tune and the incidental music for *Call the Midwife*. With a background in scoring music for both documentaries and drama, he was the perfect choice to balance the show's unique blend of fact and fiction.

Peter explains: 'Working on *Call the Midwife* I was keen, as we all were, not to produce a purely period "museum" piece. I wanted to reference the music of the time, particularly its lightness and optimism, but also to create something fresh, direct and contemporary.'

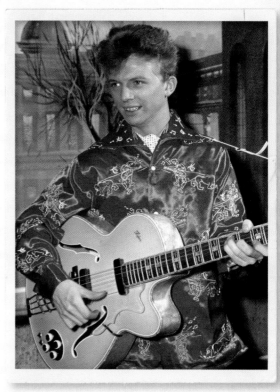

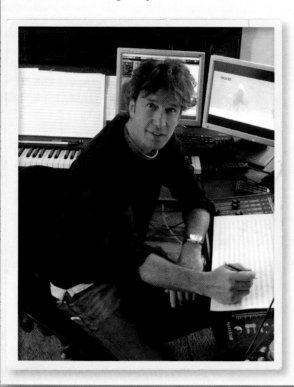

He was also keen that his orchestrations should reflect, however subtly, the tone of the original 1950s' music that features in each episode. Certain instruments and sounds struck him as appropriate as soon as he read the scripts. 'One was a certain pizzicato string sound, which you get in songs by singers such as Tommy Steele, and is very characteristic of the period. Another was a twangy, tremolo fifties' guitar sound.'

As soon as filming was under way, Peter began to develop his ideas by studying early footage and partially edited scenes. 'This always gets a few themes going,' he says, 'then I can establish a musical palette and a tone which will serve as a thread through the whole series.'

As the series took shape, Peter came up with four distinct themes. 'Among the most striking shots I saw were the wonderful images of midwives on bikes,' he remarks. 'This inspired the "biking theme" which references the string pizzicato idea, and also the slidy strings you might find in a Ricky Valence song.' Peter approached these passages in a minimalist, contemporary way, to give a more modern edge, and a sense of drive. He adds, 'Those images and this theme encapsulate more than anything for me the sense of joy, excitement and endeavour of a young Jenny starting her career in the East End.'

Next came the idea of the 'march of the heroes'. Peter explains: 'This theme was used to accompany the midwives when they were on a mission, and also over the shots of the mothers in the clinic. The pizzicato element of this also found its way into a third, crucial piece – the theme tune. Finally, there was a nostalgic piano piece. Originally, this was intended to be a theme connected to Jenny's past. However, as the show evolved, it also proved incredibly useful for the development of Chummy into a first-class midwife.'

The instruments featured also changed as work progressed. 'In the end, the guitar only gets an occasional look-in,' Peter comments. 'Although I particularly enjoyed combining it with plainchant in Episode Two of the first series.' In this sequence, Peter underscored the sight and sound of the nuns at prayer with a sequence of melancholy guitar chords. This unique combination then played over

the subsequent scenes of young prostitute Mary plying her trade near the docks. Peter explains: 'I wanted to heighten the contrast between the spiritual life at Nonnatus House, with the stark reality of the lives of ordinary people around them.'

For Peter, the highlight of the whole composing process comes at the recording sessions for the music. 'On *Call the Midwife* I am lucky enough to have a string section of the finest chamber players, a wonderful pianist, and the occasional glorious clarinettist to bring the music to life, and give it the feel which only live playing can.' He smiles and says, 'Standing in front of them, waving my arms around, as the cues I have written become music is sheer pleasure.'

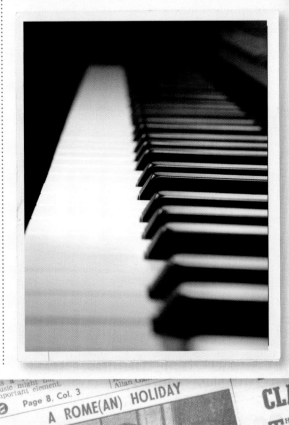

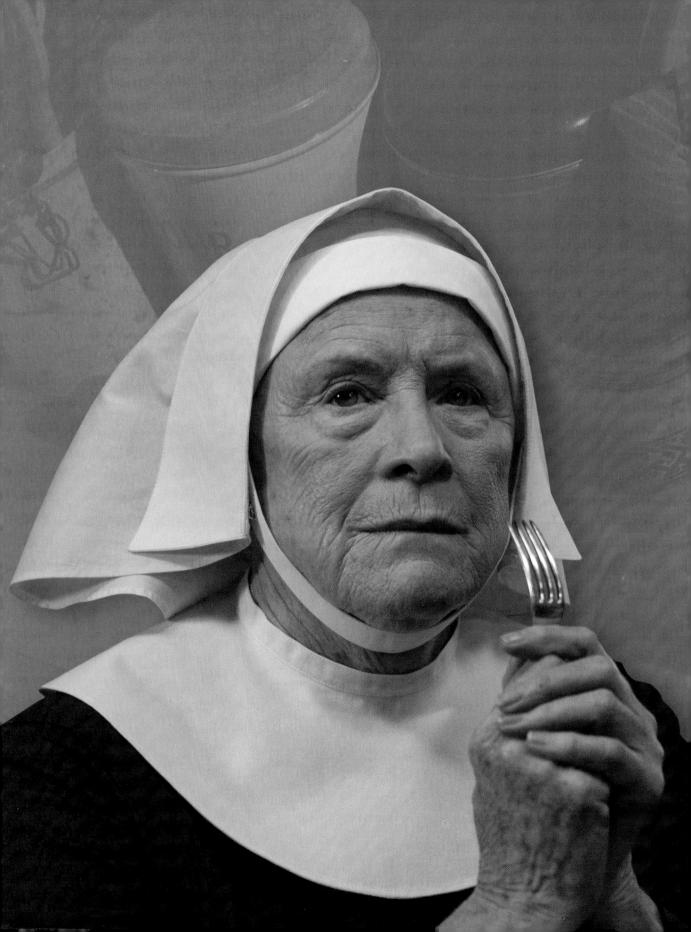

CHAPTER
7
Food

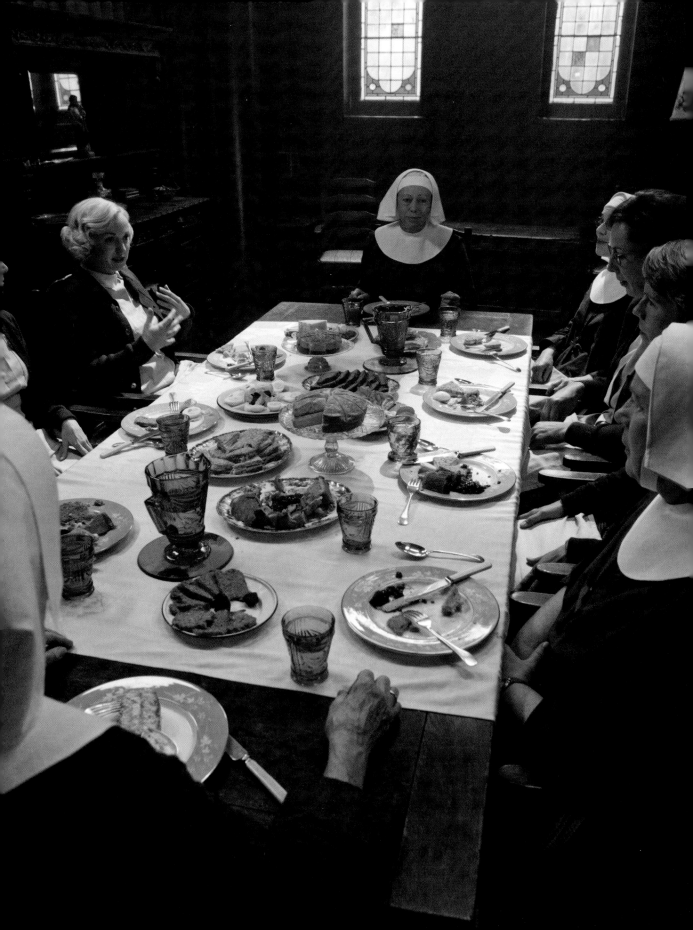

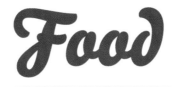

Food

'YOU MUST HAVE ANOTHER SLICE.'

Sister Monica Joan

'I'M ALMOST FULL.'

Jenny

'YOU ARE YOUNG, YOU CAN NEVER BE FILLED.
YOU HAVE AN APPETITE FOR LIFE.'

Sister Monica Joan

It was only when the first series of *Call the Midwife* aired that I realised quite how much food – and indeed drink – we had put into the script. At every turn, there seemed to be plates full of sandwiches, paper parcels full of chips, and Berylware cups full of steaming tea or Horlicks. In the opening episode of the show, Jenny Lee is ushered into Nonnatus House by Sister Monica Joan, who imperiously declares that they should 'go in search of cake'. After some sleuthing, a coconut sponge is located in a hiding place, and the mischevious nun and Jenny eat the lot. Sister Evangelina – doomed to snack on Gypsy Creams – takes some time to forgive the errant newcomer. Sweet treats are of great importance in Nonnatus House – the nurses tuck into cold bread pudding while they get drunk on sherry and play Monopoly, and Chummy frantically makes meringues when her mother comes to visit.

People started joining in, recording their TV snacks on Twitter: 'Watching #callthemidwife with a piece of chocolate cheesecake. Mmmm!' was a typical example.

Food seems to be part and parcel of the pleasure of the show, and perhaps this is entirely appropriate. After the years of wartime rationing, which ended in 1954, by the late fifties food was becoming more abundant, more convenient, more modern. It was en route to being a delight rather than merely a means of sustenance. Some found this harder to embrace than others.

The war years left their mark in two contrasting ways. On the one hand, there were women like my maternal grandmother Edith, who had raised four children while groceries were rationed and had to be queued up for. Although she was the wife of a prosperous butcher, she so struggled to vary and flavour

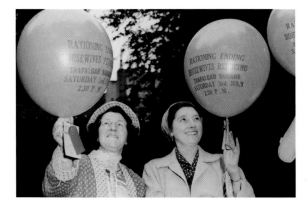

the family's meals that when he gave her the unromantic anniversary gift of a pound of onions she was beside herself with joy. Until she was 90, the shelves of Edith's walk-in larder were testament to tough times in the past – every inch of gristle and dab of cold pudding was swathed in greaseproof and kept for another day. Nothing, but nothing, was ever thrown away.

Meanwhile my parents – raised on rationed sweets in a world where bananas were only a rumour – grew up, like many of their generation, to be almost profligate with food. Meat (there were butchers on both sides of the family) was always a feature in our house – huge roasts, garlands of sausages, plates spilling over with savoury mince. And there were crumbles and pies with custard or tinned cream, and Battenburg cakes, and Tizer, and chocolate

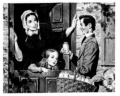

Faith has been kept

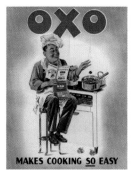

MAKES COOKING SO EASY

teacakes wrapped in foil if we were peckish between meals. Food had become an indulgence, a language, a celebration of all that was good – and the roots of this lay firmly in the fifties.

As Jennifer Worth once said to me, people might have lived in appalling housing in Poplar, but they were far from starving. During her time there, employment rates were good and wages were increasing. Meanwhile, with mechanised farming on the rise, food prices were falling and the shops replete with items that were tasty and convenient.

Ease of preparation was essential in working class homes, where kitchens were basic, fridges rare, and few women bothered with recipe books. The tinned meat product Spam – its name an abbreviation of 'spiced ham' – had grown in popularity during the War, and was eaten cold, fried or as fritters. Tinned corned beef was consumed in sandwiches or pounded into hash with onions and potatoes. Pasta was virtually unknown – Jennifer said the only time she ever came across it was in the home of Conchita Warren, who was born in Spain.

Dried goods had long been of supreme importance in cooking. Many women still baked at home, out of necessity rather than indulgence. Today, home baking is all about conspicuous consumption, but the most striking feature of post-war baking was restraint. Sandwich tins

People might have lived in appalling housing in Poplar, but they were far from starving.

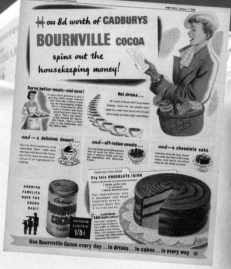

were six inches wide, not eight. Cocoa powder was used, not melted chocolate, and there were no gaudy muffins with an inch of cream cheese frosting – only delicate fairy cakes, topped with a careful circle of pale icing. There is a sweet Spartan elegance about these recipes, enhanced by the pared-down geometry of Imperial measures. Four ounces of this, two of that, a Size 1 egg. Ingredients that could be bought in bulk and stored for a long time made the pennies go further, and raisins, sultanas and currants gave heft to many a recipe.

The nuns cycle up to twenty miles per day, and feel they have earned their indulgent tea-time treats.

Bev Gerard, *Call the Midwife*'s Standby Art Director, is responsible for all the food that appears on set. 'Special cakes are commissioned from quality bakers such as Dunn's in London's Crouch End,' she reveals. 'Some just come from Waitrose, although when we needed a birthday cake for Jenny in Series Two, the girls in the Art department made it!'

The nuns cycle up to twenty miles per day, and feel they have earned their indulgent tea-time treats. The actors are very committed to representing this aspect of convent life on screen. They all tuck in with gusto, even when they must eat several scones, one after the other for the sake of continuity.

Savoury items such as meatloaf and sandwiches also feature in the series. 'We tend to buy the bits needed for food scenes and put them together ourselves based on reference photos or adverts of fifties food,' says Bev, adding, 'I think the food always brings life to the kitchen, even if it's just a jar of home made jam.'

In the kitchen of Nonnatus House, the art department have meticulously recreated a late fifties' larder. From Heinz, there are tins of Cream of Tomato soup and Baked Beans. Both had been imported into England from America since before World War One, and by the mid-twenties company founder Henry J. Heinz was boasting that he sold '57 Varieties'. Another item on the shelves that is still available today is Oxo, which supposedly gave a meal 'man appeal'. Meanwhile, Bird's Custard – a cornflour preparation invented by a man whose wife was intolerant of eggs – also earns a prominent place.

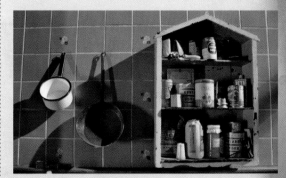

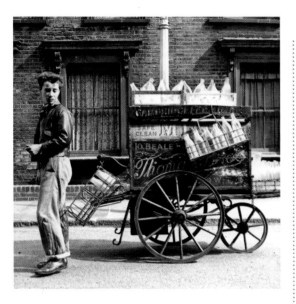

cereal, and it was the principal ingredient of the ubiquitous milk pudding, baked along with rice, semolina, macaroni, tapioca or a strange precursor to polenta called Cremola. It was also drunk by the mugful at bedtime, mixed with commercial beverage powders such as Horlicks, Ovaltine and Bournvita. These malted drinks were supposed to aid restful sleep, and Horlicks in particular was looked on as a health food. This was largely due to the success of its claims that 'Horlicks guards against night starvation' – a debilitating complaint created by the manufacturer. Fresh milk was delivered in glass bottles in the early hours of the morning, by electric float or horse-drawn cart. The empty bottles were rinsed and left to be collected and recycled, in what now appears to be a model 'green' initiative. Bakers' vans also toured the streets, as did large lorries selling the all-essential fifties' fizzy drinks.

Like dining, shopping was an entirely different experience. High streets traditionally hosted a baker, a butcher, a fishmonger and perhaps a Co-Op store with staff at every counter.

Greengrocers dealt in strictly seasonal produce – long before such limitations were thought smart – with prices daubed in whitewash on the windows every morning.

Bird's Custard had, of course, to be mixed with milk, which was the prop and mainstay of the national diet in the mid-20th century.

Life must have been grim for the lactose intolerant. Even during the War the adult ration of milk was 3 pints per week, which would easily sustain an individual in the present day, and yet this was deemed a scarcely tolerable hardship. By the middle of the fifties, the brakes were well and truly off – milk was available fresh, sterilised, powdered, tinned, condensed, evaporated, as cream or ice cream and in custard.

It was poured over

Fresh milk was delivered in glass bottles in the early hours of the morning, by electric float or cart, and bakers' vans toured the streets.

Desiccated coconut was a popular cake ingredient in the fifties. My cousin Jenny recalls a speciality coconut cake made by my paternal granny, who was known as Mamma. Jenny loathed it, but the grandsons loved it, so to her chagrin it appeared every week. Interestingly, there were two versions of the recipe. One – a layer cake sandwiched with buttercream – was kept for high days and holidays. The other was plain, restrained, and seen with greater frequency, topped only with a simple strip of peel. We featured the richer version of the coconut cake in the opening episode of *Call the Midwife*. It would be prettier to look at, and its disappearance more likely to cause ructions.

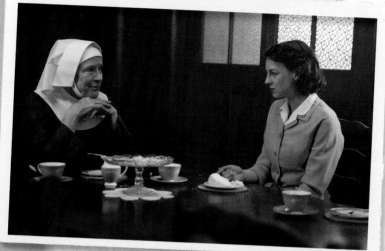

RECIPE

MAMMA'S COCONUT CAKE

6 oz unsalted butter
(at room temperature)
6 oz caster sugar
4 medium eggs, beaten
8 oz self-raising flour
1 tsp baking powder
3 oz desiccated coconut
2 tbsp whole milk
2 strips of candied lemon peel

Pre-heat the oven to 160ºC/140ºC fan/Gas mark 4.

Line the base and sides of an 8 in round cake tin with baking parchment.

Place the butter and sugar in a bowl and beat until pale and fluffy. In a separate bowl, mix the flour with the baking powder and desiccated coconut. Beat the eggs into the butter and sugar mixture a spoonful at a time, then stir in the dry ingredients. Stir the milk into the cake mixture and spoon it into the prepared cake tin. Smooth out the mixture gently with a spatula and place the peel gently on top.

Bake for 1¼ hours until golden brown. Remove and leave to cool on a wire rack before turning it out. It should have a domed top with little cracks that hold the peel.

COCONUT LAYER CAKE

INGREDIENT.—¼ lb. of desiccated coconut, ½ lb. of castor sugar, ½ lb. of margarine, ¾ lb. of flour, 1½ teaspoon-fuls of cream of tartar, ½ flat teaspoon-ful of carbonate of soda, 3 eggs, milk.

FOR THE BUTTER ICING.—12 oz. of icing sugar, vanilla flavouring, 6 oz. of butter, desiccated coconut.

METHOD.—Grease a cake-tin and line with gerased paper in the usual way.

Sieve the flour with the cream of tartar and carbonate of soda. Whisk up the eggs. Cream the fat and sugar. Gradually stir in the flour, etc., and coconut alternately with the eggs, and some milk as required.

Mix all together and beat well, put into the cake-tin and bake in a moderately hot oven for about one hour and a quarter, lessening the heat as the cake begins to brown.

When cooked, turn out carefully and leave on a sieve until cold.

TO MAKE THE ICING.—Roll the lumps out of the icing sugar and rub it through a fine sieve.

Add the butter and beat both to a cream.

Flavour with vanilla.

TO ICE THE CAKE.—Split the cake into three and spread some of the icing between each layer, then sand-wich together again.

Spread a layer of icing on the top and all round the sides of the cake, then coat with desiccated coconut.

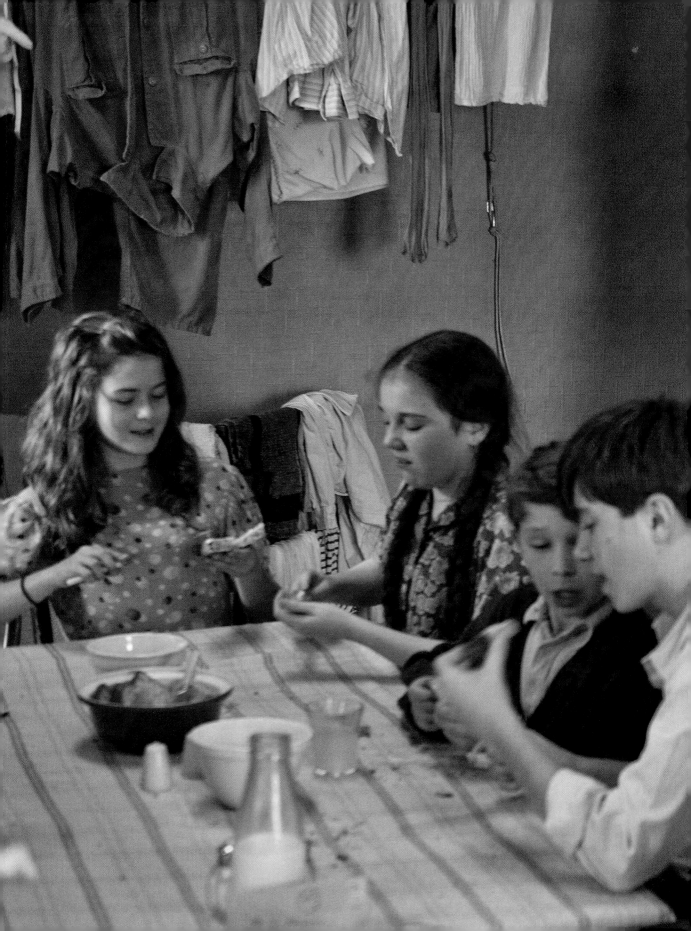

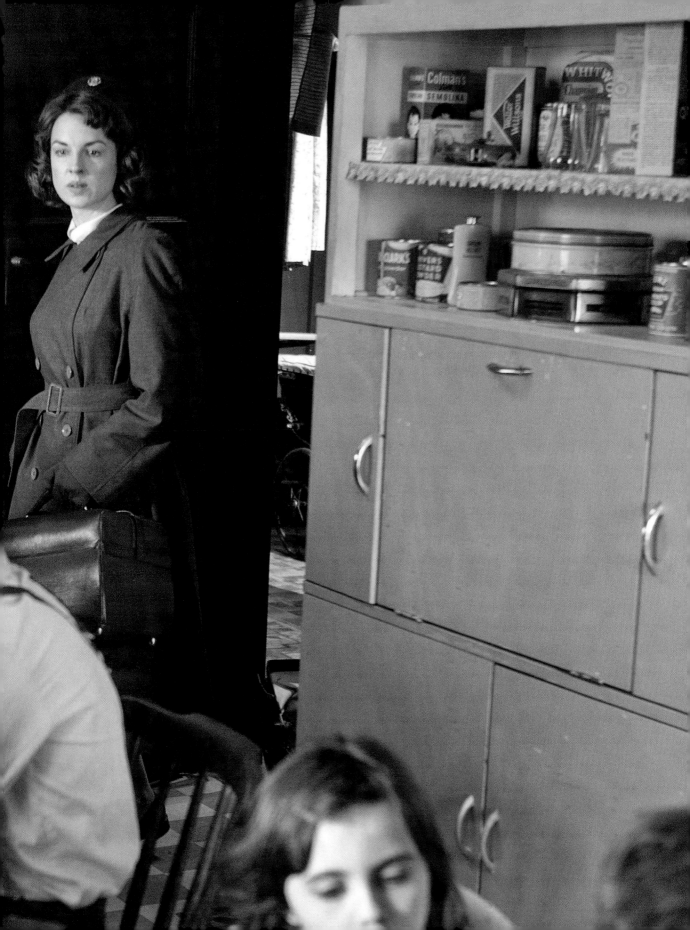

HOT GOBLIN'S FAMOUS SCOTCH EGGS

8 eggs
Sunflower oil, for shallow frying
1 leek, trimmed and finely chopped
6 pork sausages, squeezed out of the skins
1 tbsp Dijon mustard
Salt and freshly ground black pepper
3 tbsp plain flour
200 g breadcrumbs

Bring a pan of water to the boil, add 6 of the eggs and boil them for 5 minutes (the yolks are best if they are slightly runny). Drain the eggs, rinse them under cold water and leave in a bowl of cold water to cool completely. Peel carefully.

Heat a small amount of the oil in a large frying pan over a medium heat, add the leek and fry for about 10 minutes until soft. Tip into a bowl and add the sausage meat and mustard, and season with salt and pepper. Mix together thoroughly, then divide into six balls.

Flatten a ball of sausage meat in the palm of your hand, place an egg in the middle of the flattened ball and then wrap the sausage meat around the egg. Repeat with the other balls and eggs.

Beat the remaining 2 eggs in a shallow bowl. Put the flour in another bowl and the breadcrumbs in a third. Dip each coated egg in flour, then in the beaten egg and, finally, the breadcrumbs. Place on a baking sheet and chill for 30 minutes.

Heat a pan of oil (no more than one-third full but deep enough to hold the eggs) over a medium heat until a cube of bread browns in a minute. Gently lower in the eggs, in batches if necessary, and cook for about 5 minutes until they are golden. Lift the eggs out of the pan one by one with a slotted spoon and place on kitchen paper to drain. Serve warm, standing in the rain (in the middle of summer) on the *Call the Midwife* set in Mill Hill.

The Hot Goblin catering team feed 80 to 100 cast and crew every day.

STUFFED BUTTERNUT SQUASH

1 butternut squash, halved lengthways
Salt and freshly ground black pepper
½ tsp paprika
3 tbsp snipped chives
3 tbsp crème fraîche
2 thick slices of white bread, crumbled into breadcrumbs
Generous knob of butter, melted
25 g Parmesan cheese, grated

Preheat the oven to 200°C/180°C fan/Gas mark 6.

Use a spoon to scoop out the seeds from the butternut squash halves. Season the shells with salt and pepper and put in a roasting tin that is half full of water. Cover with foil and bake in the oven for about 40 minutes until the squash is tender, but not collapsing.

Drain off the water. Transfer the squash to a board and leave until cool enough to handle. Scrape most of the flesh into a bowl, leaving a thin border of flesh on the skin. Return the squash shells to the roasting tin and set aside.

Add the paprika, chives and crème fraîche to the squash flesh, mix thoroughly and season to taste. Pile the mixture into the squash shells. Mix the breadcrumbs with the butter and Parmesan and sprinkle on top, and bake for about 15 minutes until lightly browned.

Fruit and vegetables occupied a very different place in the nation's affections in the fifties. If there was anything you fancied, you had to grab it while you could – strawberries, for example, were available for about eight weeks per year, and English cherries for perhaps a fortnight. Oranges, apples and bananas were in the shops year round, but treated almost as ornaments and displayed in special bowls on the sideboard. Grapes were for the sick.

Allotments and backyard vegetable plots remained popular long after the War was over. In *Call the Midwife*, we see the nuns growing their own salad stuffs and cabbages in the cloister garden, while Frank and Peggy cherish a little vine outside their prefab. Nowadays, soil on vegetables is seen as pleasing proof of authenticity, and often as a sign that the item is organic. But in the fifties, mud was just mud and nothing to do with Farmers' Markets – everything was sold in its natural state as no farmer had the means to wash it. Perhaps it was this reminder of food's earthy origins that provoked the habit of extended cooking. Most vegetables were routinely boiled for forty minutes, with plenty of salt, and it wasn't uncommon to go to church and leave the carrots and swede on a low light.

However, the age of the supermarket was dawning and it would radically alter the way that people shopped. When it arrived, the self-service model wasn't instantly popular. Sceptics – perhaps correctly – saw it as a speedy way to spend a lot of money. Wire baskets and trolleys were introduced in an effort to limit thefts, and this symbol of suspicion provoked a lot of tutting. But while in 1950 a scant fifty supermarkets were in existence, across the decade the number increased tenfold.

Recipes from the kitchen of the Community of St John the Divine

Like the nuns of Nonnatus House, the Sisters of the Community of St John the Divine are keen cooks, who bake their own bread daily, grow their own produce, and delight in sharing a Miracle Pudding with their guests – the 'miracle' being a heavenly molten layer of rich butterscotch sauce.

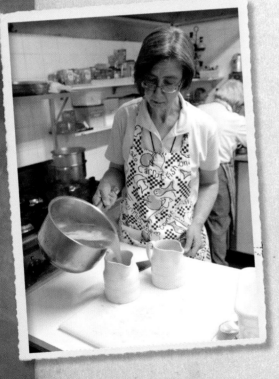

RECIPE

ST JOHN'S WHOLEMEAL BREAD

1 tsp runny honey or caster sugar
300 ml warm water
1 sachet (7 g) fast action yeast
500 g wholemeal flour
1½ tsp salt
2 tsp dark brown sugar
1 tbsp light olive or sunflower oil,
plus extra for greasing

Place the honey in a measuring jug with 50 ml warm water, stir to melt the honey, then sprinkle in the yeast. Place the jug in a warm place until the yeast mixture is frothy and the mixture has risen in the jug.

Meanwhile, put the flour, salt and brown sugar into a microwaveable bowl and heat in the microwave on Medium for 45 seconds, to warm the ingredients.

Put the warmed flour into an electric mixer bowl, add the oil and mix using a dough hook. Add the frothy yeast mixture and mix, then gradually add the warm water (the mixture may not need all of it) until the dough sticks to the hook and leaves the sides of the bowl. If the dough looks a bit wet, add a small amount of flour. While the dough is mixing, grease a 2 lb loaf tin.

Turn the dough out onto a floured board and knead until smooth. Shape it and place it in the greased tin. Cover the tin with a clean damp tea towel and leave in a warm place for 30–45 minutes until the dough has doubled in size. *Preheat the oven to 230°C/210°C fan/Gas mark 8.*

Remove the tea towel and bake for 30–35 minutes. The loaf should sound hollow when tapped underneath. Lower the heat of the oven to 150°C/130°C fan/Gas mark 5. Return the loaf to the oven (without the tin) with the bottom of the loaf facing upwards for about 5 minutes. This will help the loaf crust firm up. Remove and leave to cool on a wire rack.

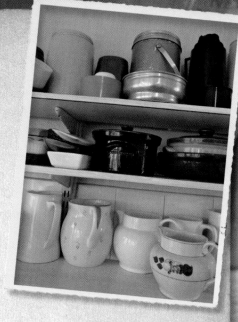

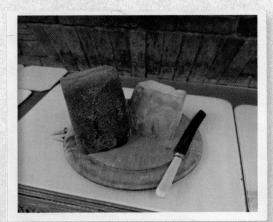

RECIPE

ST JOHN'S MIRACLE PUDDING

150 g self-raising flour
150 g margarine or unsalted butter, chopped into small pieces
about 2 tbsp milk
110 g sultanas
110 g soft brown sugar

Preheat the oven to 180°C/160°C fan/Gas mark 4. Grease a 15 cm ovenproof dish (8 cm deep).

Put the flour into a bowl and rub in half of the margarine. Add a little of the milk and mix to a stiff dough; add the sultanas, and some more milk if necessary.

Put the sugar and remaining margarine into a small saucepan and add 400 ml (14 fl oz) of water. Gently heat until the sugar and margarine have melted and formed a smooth butterscotch sauce (this is the miracle bit!).

Put the dough in the ovenproof dish, pour over the sugar sauce and bake for 35–40 minutes until risen and golden.

The on-set caterers lay out the food on a long buffet table, where everyone — from electricians to leading ladies — rubs shoulders and chats as they help themselves to lunch.

Ready-cooked food was always popular in Poplar. The most enduring speciality was pie and mash. Originally, the pies contained eels, which could be easily acquired from the polluted River Thames. Later, they featured meat, usually minced beef or lamb. For the truly hungry, the pies were served with mashed potato and a thin parsley gravy, known as liquor.

Eels were also sold cold, preserved in gelatine. In the first series of *Call the Midwife*, Chummy – who had bonded with her boyfriend PC Noakes over fish and chips – expresses dislike of jellied eels, which called to mind the salmon-in-aspic she had suffered as a debutante. I created a sneaky date for the uniformed couple at an East End whelk stall, only to be told, after the whelk stall had been built, that Miranda Hart was unable to eat seafood. The Art Department came to our rescue with tiny cut-out chicken 'whelks'.

For the cast of *Call the Midwife*, food remains central to their daily on-set experience, thanks to caterers who produce a cooked breakfast and a hot lunch every day. The menu might include a choice of roast lamb, puy lentil casserole and cod and prawn saganaki, as well as a selection of cheeses and desserts.

'This is like restaurant cooking for the same people every single day for six months, delivered out of a trailer,' Christopher, the owner, explains. 'The food has to be as good as you can possibly make it. It must be something for everybody to look forward to.' Along with chef Paul Creasey, Christopher feeds between 80 and 120 people each day.

Stuffed butternut squash is an enduring favourite (see page 196 for the recipe), and we were once all very taken with a massive ham en croute. However, dishes are chosen for practical reasons, as well as their appeal. The food Christopher chooses mustn't spoil if left standing. 'We have to be able to hold back the meals if the cast and crew aren't ready. The most important thing is the filming, that is why we are here.'

However, one of the most enjoyable aspects of the on-set food at *Call the Midwife* is simply the way it is served. Unusually for a film set, most of it is laid out on a long buffet table, where everyone – from electricians to leading ladies – rubs shoulders and chats as they help themselves to lunch. It makes the experience not just a refuelling pit stop, but a place of social interaction.

The dining room in Nonnatus House fulfils a similar function in the series. As executive producer Pippa Harris notes, 'When the nuns and the nurses gather for high tea, there's huge pleasure to be had from the meatloaf and the scones with cream and strawberries. But it's also where they share their news, and stories of the past. It's where they make plans for the future.' Pippa believes the power of these scenes lies not so much in what is on the table, as in what happens around it. 'The women of Nonnatus House are not just eating, they are communicating – like a family. And, in this day and age, that seems a very special thing.'

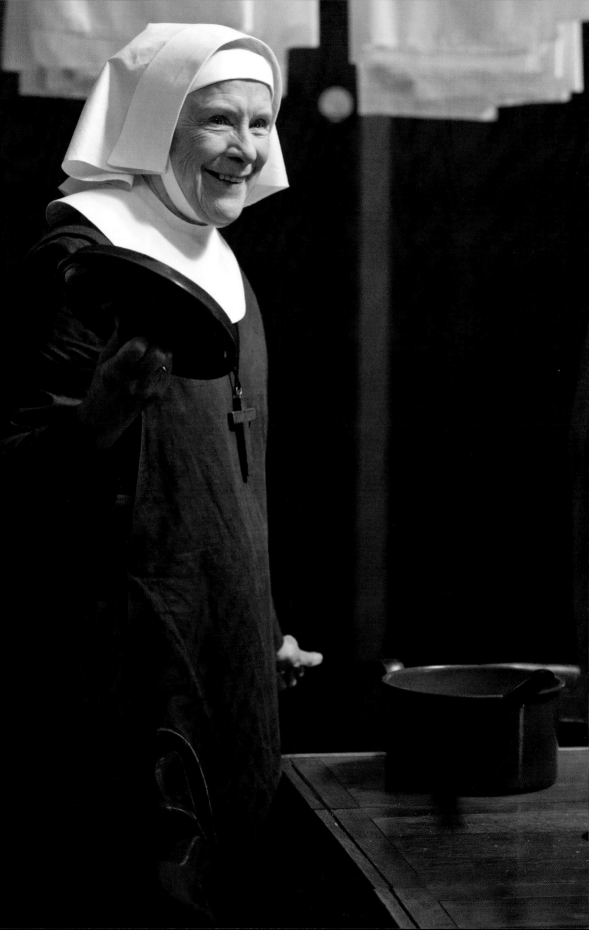

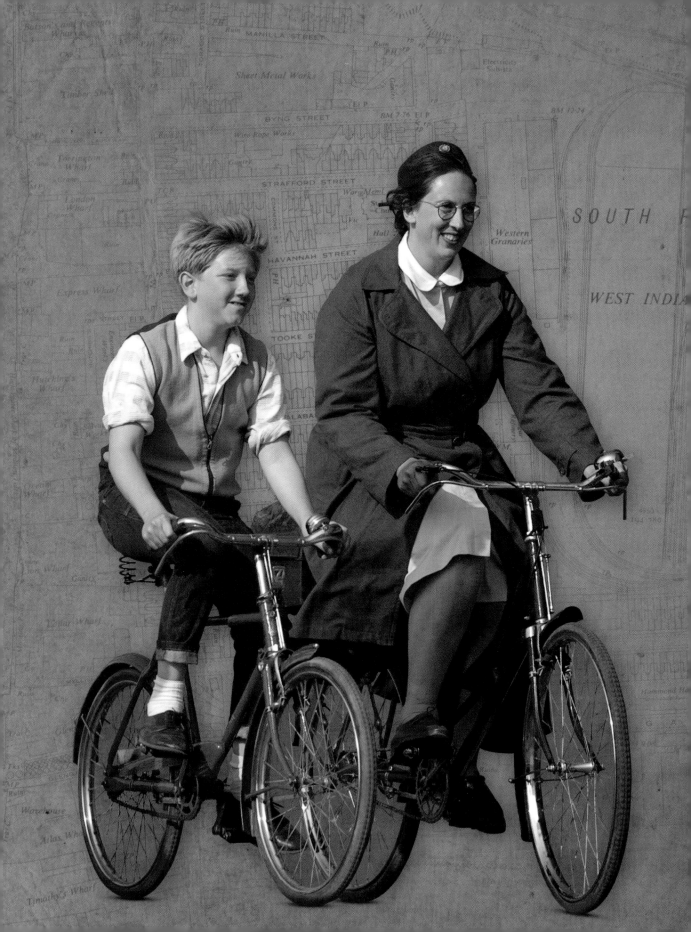

CHAPTER
8
STREET LIFE

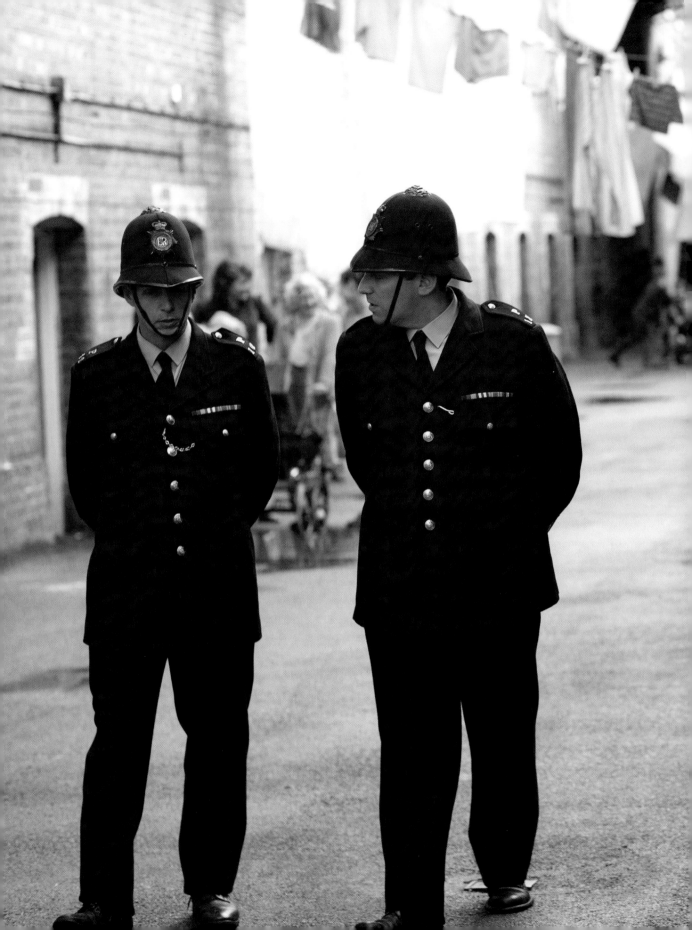

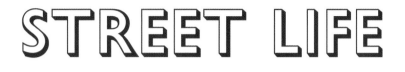

STREET LIFE

'JESUS WASHED THE FEET OF THE APOSTLES.'
SISTER MONICA JOAN

'I BET THEY HADN'T BEEN TRAMPING ALL OVER
THE BACK STREETS OF POPLAR, WALKING IN DOG
MUCK, AND MOTOR OIL, AND WORSE.'
SISTER EVANGELINA

When I first started writing the scripts for *Call the Midwife*, Jennifer Worth adored the thought of seeing fifties' Poplar brought to life on screen. 'How will you do it?' she would ask. 'How will you show the West Ferry swing bridge? And the bombed out buildings, and the ships going by at the end of the street?' The honest answer was that I did not know.

Almost nothing of Jennifer's Poplar now remains. Felled like a forest in the slum-clearance of the sixties, it has been replaced by the high-rise community now known as Tower Hamlets. Scarcely a street from Jennifer's time still stands, and since the advent of container shipping even the docks have changed beyond all recognition.

As ever, I was worried that Jennifer might be disappointed. But I had reckoned without the genius of television.

From an early stage in the proceedings, Eve Stewart, our production designer, and the producer Hugh Warren were on the hunt for potential filming venues. One of the buildings in which we film – St Joseph's Seminary in Mill Hill – provided a perfect exterior for *Call the Midwife's* Nonnatus House, and Eve dressed the forecourt with rubble to create a standing 'street' set that brilliantly conjured up the bombsites of the time.

However, the Historic Dockyard at Chatham, Kent, was possibly their greatest find – a vast, open-air museum, replete with Victorian and Georgian warehouses, courtyards and alleyways. It also provides some stupendous river frontage and features a working dock railway. Nevertheless, it took dedicated work to turn this very specific location into Jennifer's remembered streetscape.

> *'There really was no litter in the streets. It's one of the most striking things about the archive photos of the time. People had nothing to throw away.'*

PHILIPPA LOWTHORPE
Principal Director

Like most of the creative brains on *Call the Midwife*, Eve finds a rich source of inspiration in archive photographs and film. She pored over pictures of East India Docks in the fifties. In addition to fleshing out the bigger picture – showing the scale and sweep of the dockland skyline – these offered up numberless small details. Barrows full of sheepskins en route to the wool warehouse, faded advertisements painted on brick, and the lines of washing strung between tenements all play their part in the set design. The latter are not only authentic to the period, but also add colour and movement to the scene.

Chris Seager, our Director of Photography, adds his own brand of lighting magic to the streetscape. The buildings in Chatham are tall, and cast long shadows, while the riverside sunshine is unreliable. If there is a golden glow surrounding children at play, or nurses on their bikes, this is often entirely because of his expertise.

While the series is on air, old Poplar lives again for one fleeting hour each week. But, having grown from a small hamlet in the early 1800s, it is an area that experienced wave after wave of change throughout the 20th century and into the 21st.

The first alterations to the Victorian townscape came with a devastating air attack during World War One. On 13 June 1917, a school in Upper North Street was flattened in a Zeppelin raid. Eighteen children were killed, the majority aged under six. Fifteen of them were buried in a single grave in the East London cemetery.

The demolition work begun by Kaiser Bill continued during the twenties, with the first notable programme of slum clearance. The local council, which took pride in its Socialist leanings, remarked in its 1927 annual report:

'Thanks to the well-nigh superhuman efforts of the Council, no less than three hundred houses have already been constructed under the Housing Acts, and it is anticipated that two hundred more will be erected this year. Such a record, in a densely populated district, is one of which any borough might well be proud.'

The council was also extremely proud of facilities for the borough's inhabitants. By the mid-twenties two former army huts had been adapted to provide more than forty 'slipper baths' for the use of the general public. Since few had bathrooms at home, there was no shame in using these facilities. Indeed, it was deemed a mark of respectability to be seen heading off for your ablutions with your towel. In the same era, there were five municipal laundry houses dotted around Poplar, all widely patronised.

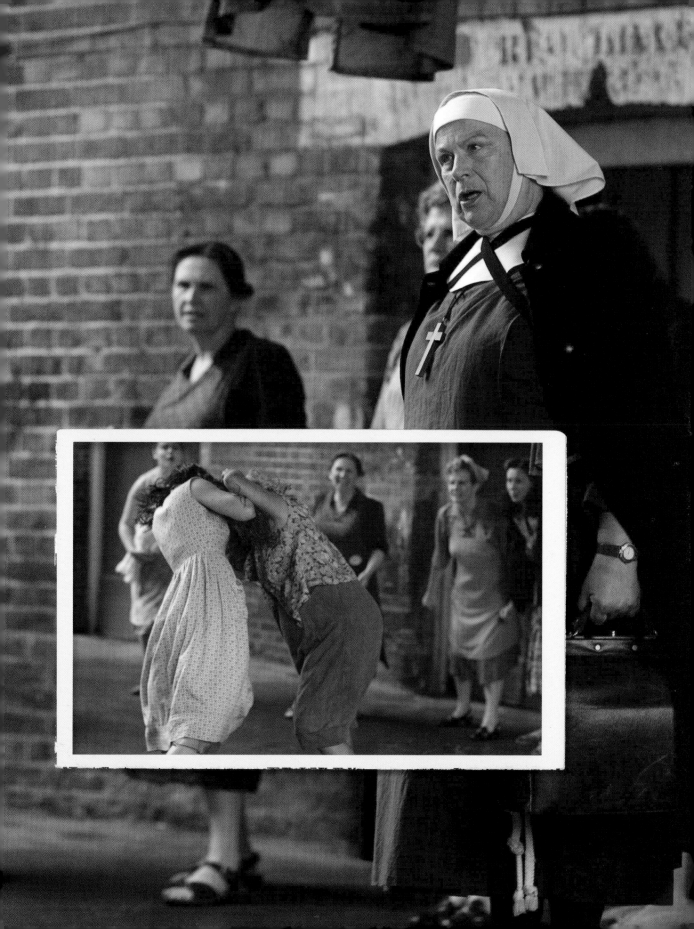

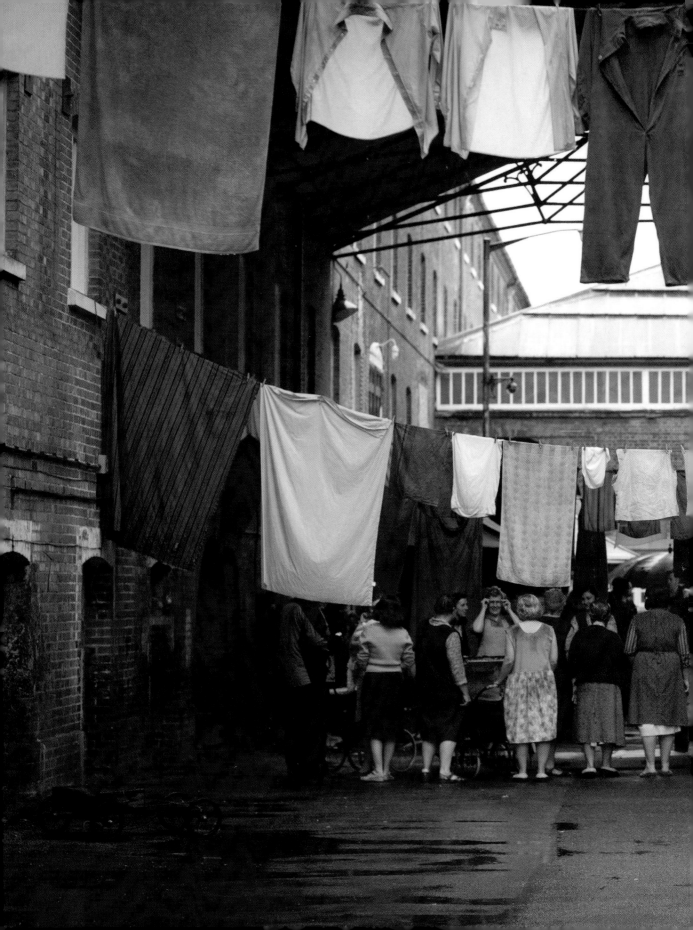

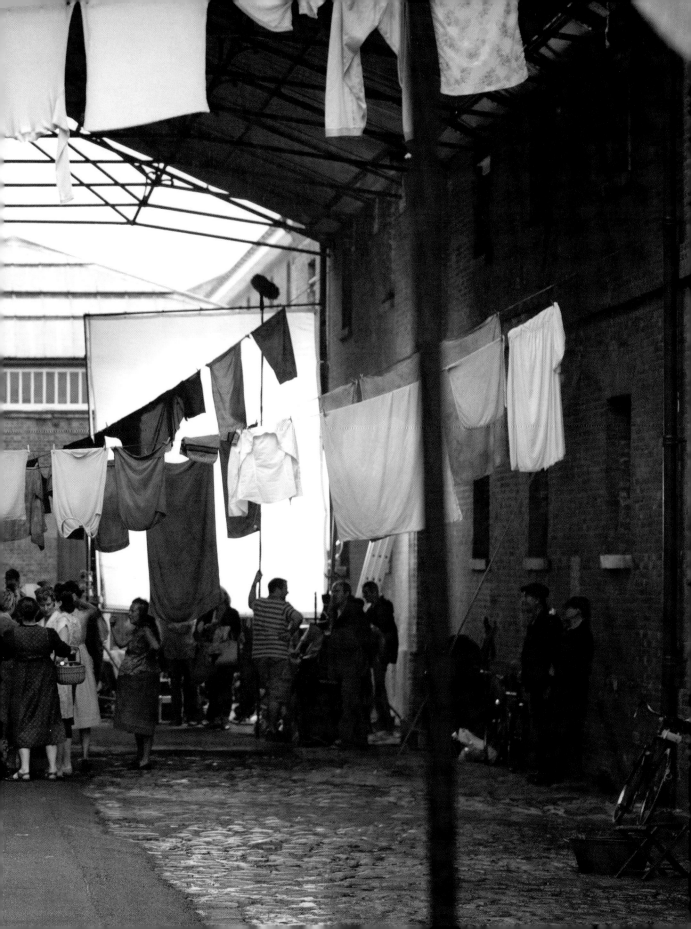

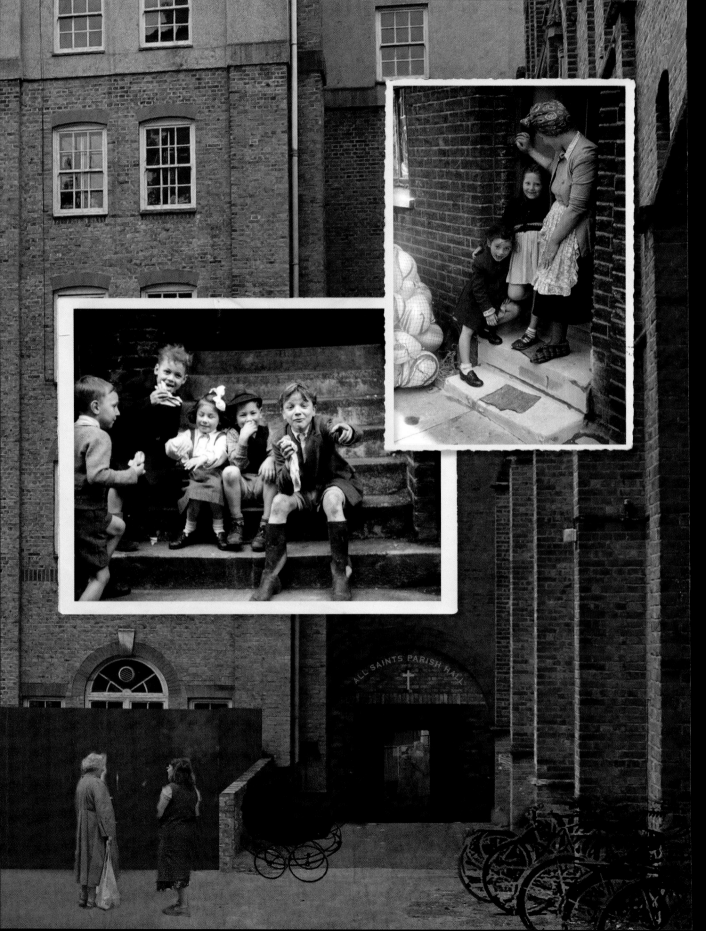

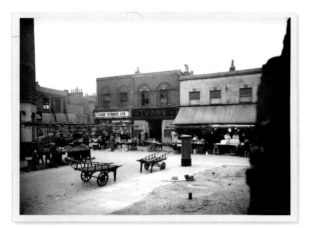

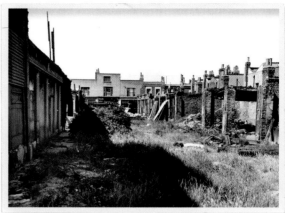

One of the interesting things about the public response to *Call the Midwife* was the way the opinion of the street scenes was polarised along class lines. Middle-class commentators thought the streets were all too clean, and those with working class roots said that they weren't clean enough.

Director Philippa Lowthorpe insists, 'There really was no litter in the streets. It's one of the most striking things about the archive photos of the time. But, if you think about it, where would the litter have come from? People had nothing to throw away. There was no fast food on sale and little in the way of domestic rubbish.'

In addition, across the middle of the 20th century, a high priority was placed on keeping public places spick and span, and it wasn't just because of civic pride.

According to research carried out by the London School of Economics, Poplar was the poorest corner of London at the start of the 1930s. As national unemployment levels soared, the council did its best to alleviate the crisis by expanding its public works. Roads were paved, swimming pools built, and 54 roads lined with newly planted trees. Meanwhile, street cleaning assumed a hitherto unknown priority. Some 5,000 men were engaged to wield brooms and dustcarts, drawing a weekly wage from the council at a time when jobs, food and shelter

were all hard to come by. Many men kept these jobs for life and took immense pride in their work.

And then ... along came Hitler. The docks were an obvious target for the Luftwaffe as they were crucial to Britain's war effort and easily visible from the air. Poplar and the surrounding areas were pounded incessantly during the Blitz. The suffering of the residents was so intense that when Buckingham Palace received a direct hit in 1940, demolishing its chapel, the then Queen Elizabeth remarked that she was glad. 'I now feel I can look the East End in the face,' she said.

The spirit of the local people remained famously unbroken, and in May 1945 VE day was celebrated with street parties across the district. Bunting was strung between boarded-up buildings, and trestle tables full of sandwiches lined up in the open air. Children in fancy dress ran egg-and-spoon races on the bomb sites, but East Enders had paid a high price for Britain's victory. Terrace after terrace had been bombarded into dust, and survivors forced into the housing that remained. Extended families 'bunked in' with one another, and young married couples had no choice but to live with their parents, even after babies started to arrive. In 1953, the Coronation saw another wave of parties in the street – but the flags and fairy cakes concealed real, rising distress on the accommodation front.

RECREATING THE DOCKS

Visitors to the set at Chatham's historic dockyard are always surprised by the large, flat, bright green screens that stud the backdrop. Carefully positioned to blot out any eyesores, these are the first building blocks in the complex process of computer-generated imagery (CGI). The six episodes of Series One featured more than a hundred enhanced visual effects, including 3D models of boats, cranes, barges and cargo. Environmental effects such as fog and smoke added further period realism.

'Visual effects are often associated with explosive in-your-face images, but *Call the Midwife* was an opportunity for us to illustrate how subtle interventions throughout the film can add reality to period drama,' says Grant Hewlett, Visual Effects Supervisor.

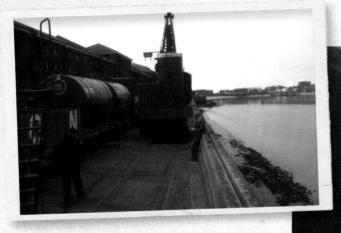

When all earthly tricks fail, CGI can create cranes with dangling cargo nets, seagulls that fly, water that ripples and a sun that moves across the heavens.

3) The third stage is 'dressing the set' (right). All the computer-built assets are laid on top of the original filmed images. The visual details are fine-tuned and animation is applied. Finally, the lighting is finessed. A sophisticated computer programme uses a technique called 'raytracing' to recreate the shift of light and shadows between surfaces. Every wavelet in the River Thames needs a ripple and all the terraced houses have to differ from their neighbours.

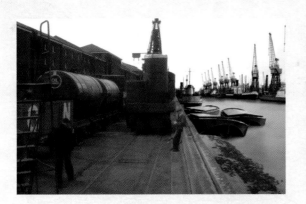

1) *The first step in the complex process of CGI is computer modelling, a geometric building exercise that creates an object on the screen in block form, providing a framework.*

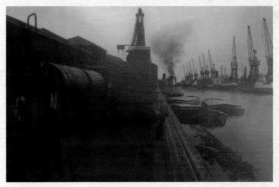

2) *Then comes 'texturing', in which any material – be it natural (such as water) or man-made (such as brick) – can be created on the screen.*

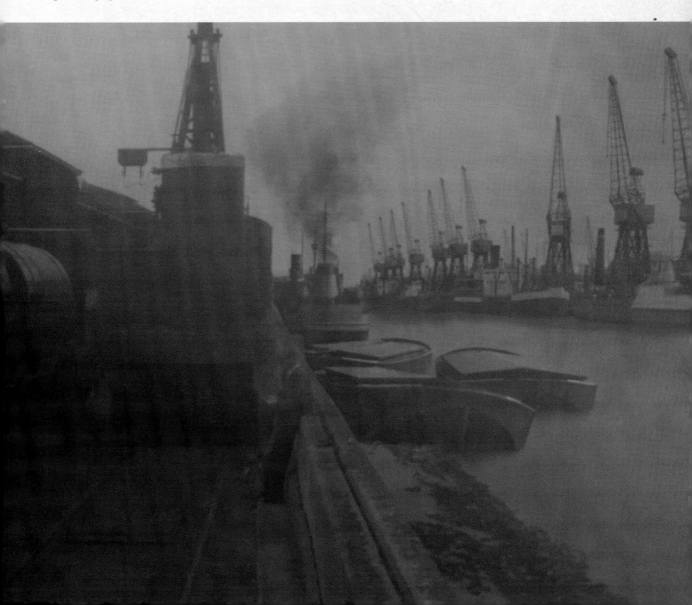

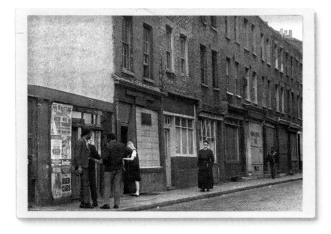

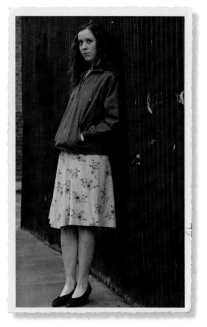

Cable Street in the 1950s, an area notorious for its brothels and all-night cafés.

By the late 1950s, when Jennifer Worth arrived in Poplar, the situation was at crisis point.

Rows of prefabricated homes, erected as a temporary measure, were starting to feel permanent, and the bombsites had become the haunt of meths drinkers. Nevertheless, ambitious town planners saw the area as a blank canvas. Gradually, new estates sprang up, changing the appearance of Poplar irrevocably. However, against all odds, the district's neighbourly spirit endured – and it was at its most apparent where childbirth was concerned.

Sister Teresa French – who, as a nun, worked alongside Jennifer Worth – has recalled how she was sent to inspect a home to see if it was suitable for a baby to be delivered there. She found it filthy and devoid of all necessities. The question was not just where the baby would be born, but how it might be cared for afterwards. She left the premises in utter despair, only to be stopped by one of the woman's neighbours, who had seen the extent of the problem.

'Don't worry, Sister,' she said. 'We'll make sure you get everything you need.' When Sister Teresa returned, the community had rallied round – bed sheets, fuel, a cot and baby clothes had been donated in abundance.

Jennifer always spoke warmly of the respect the nuns and the nurses received as they went about their rounds. Their uniforms set them apart, and because their work was valued, no nurse or nun ever had their cycle stolen, even in areas where policemen walked in pairs for their own safety.

In Series One, Jenny becomes drawn into an unusual friendship with pregnant Mary (played by Amy McAllister), who had been trafficked into prostitution in a Turkish café. Just 15 years old, Mary is first seen seeking clients near the river. Prior to the Street Offences Act in 1959, prostitutes were not forbidden to solicit openly, and were a common sight in certain areas of London.

Abused throughout her short life, Mary remains in thrall to her pimp, Zakir (played by Darwin Shaw), even after she flees the café. In an attempt to understand the pressures on the fragile girl, Jenny creeps through the alleyways of Cable Street, peering into the windows of a strip-tease club. This, for her, is a new and disturbing London – shopsoiled, sleazy and beyond her comprehension.

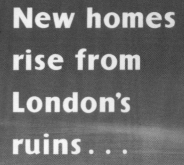

New homes rise from London's ruins...

SEE LONDON'S NEW NEIGHBOURHOOD GROWING

LANSBURY · POPLAR

Admission to neighbourhood free

Special enclosure, show house and flat, 1'6 — children 5-15 half price: children under 5 not admitted

For times of opening see newspapers

WATER BUS TO WEST INDIA DOCK PIER, AND THENCE BY BUS—OR BUS FROM ALDGATE EAST UNDERGROUND STATION

1951

Printed in Great Britain for H.M. Stationery Office by Sanders Phillips & Co., Ltd.
Prepared by London Press Exchange for Festival of Britain 1951   2 Savoy Court, London, W.C.2.

Although the East End had a rising problem with organised crime – by the late fifties the Kray Twins were already running lines in hijacking, robbery and arson – innocent bystanders generally went unmolested. Nationwide, violent crimes numbered 11,000 per year – forty years later the figure had swollen to 250,000. By day, the streets were busy with milkmen, coalmen and insurance men making house calls. Avon ladies were doing brisk business, while the rag and bone man (usually in a horse-drawn cart) remained a feature of the streetscape. Postmen made two deliveries a day, and children played in the road from dawn until dusk.

Girls loved to skip, often using long lengths of washing line stretched across the street. Their skipping games were complex, accompanied by songs whose precise lyrics varied from district to district. For boys, a leather or plastic football was a highly prized toy. Games were played in the street, with jumpers for goalposts. Even in the days of horse-drawn transport, children and traffic made for a dangerous mix. With the rise of the motor van and car, casualties grew. In 1938, taking inspiration from an earlier US law, the British government passed the Street Playgrounds Bill. This enabled local authorities to close streets to traffic between 8am and sunset, so that children could play in safety. By the late fifties, there were more than 700 play streets in England and Wales.

It was such a caring and farsighted law, that it now seems rather sad that Play Streets have been all but forgotten – and ironic that when the scheme was at its height in the 1950s, the average London street had only five cars parked on it. Indeed, private vehicle ownership was so rare that it wasn't thought necessary to invent the parking meter until 1958.

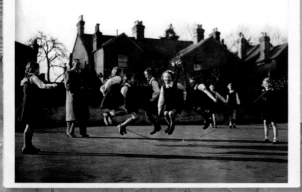

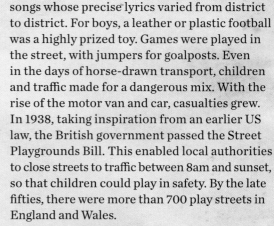

'REHEARSING A FORCEPS DELIVERY WITH A PAIR OF SALAD SERVERS. AND, SEEING CHILD EXTRAS ON A GO-KART THAT WAS EXACTLY THE SAME AS ONE I PLAYED ON AS A CHILD.'

Stephen McGann
DR TURNER

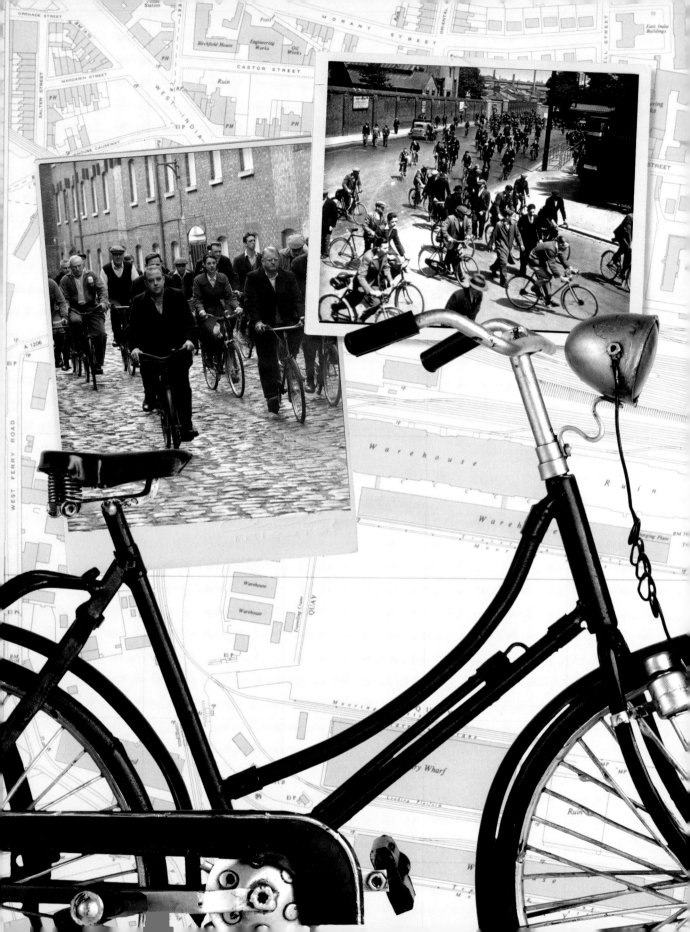

What does Call the Midwife mean to you?

'I LOVE A GOOD BIKE RIDE, ALTHOUGH IT IS A BIT DIFFERENT WITH A HEAVY MEDICAL PACK ON THE BACK.'

Laura Main
SISTER BERNADETTE

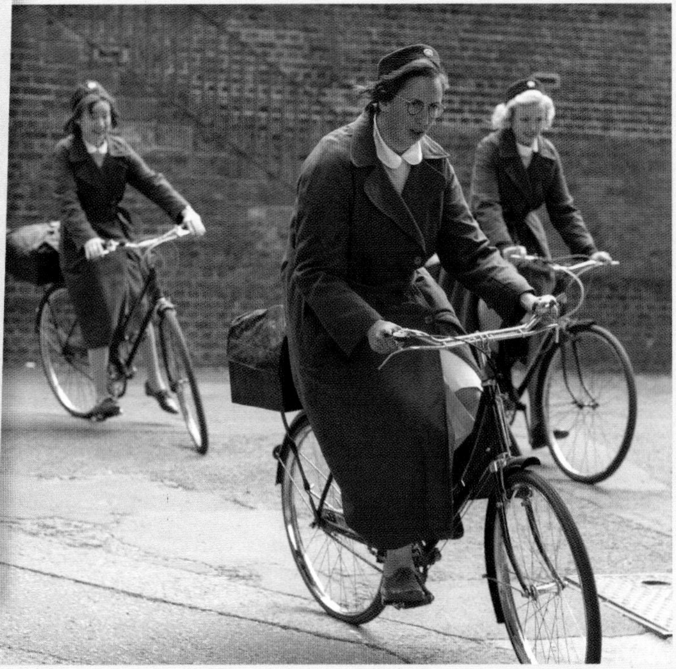

The Sisters and the single-gear 'safety bike' were a match made in heaven.

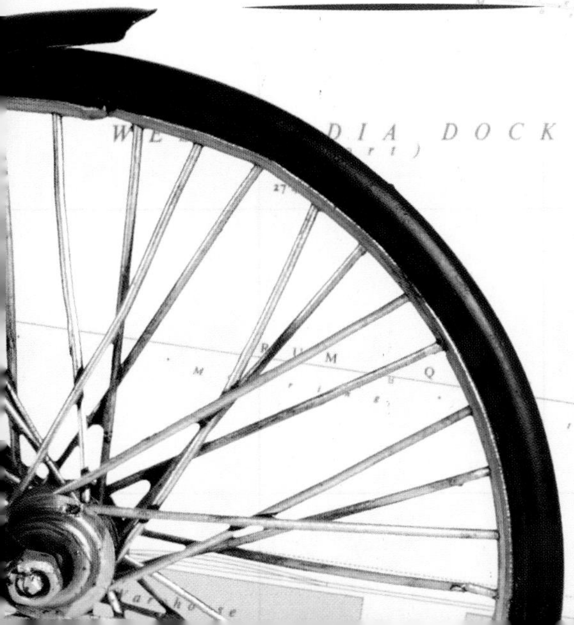

Factory workers, dockers, railway staff and numerous others relied on bikes to transport them to work. The 'safety bike', with its single gear and two equal-sized wheels, had made its first appearance in 1885. It was round about this time that the nursing nuns of the Order of St John the Divine first made links with the East End. And the Sisters and the bike were a match made in heaven – especially after the invention of the pneumatic tyre three years later. This made cycling both speedier and marginally more comfortable, but there were no further improvements for several decades.

The cast of *Call the Midwife* have reason to rue this. Pam Ferris almost flinches when recalling a particularly gruelling day's filming down at Chatham dockyard. 'I do not recommend riding an old boneshaker on not just ordinary old cobbles but very, very deep cobbles with big

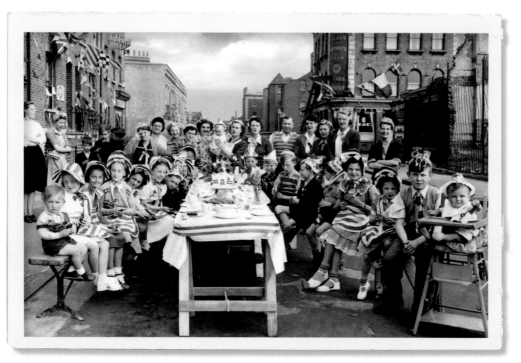

A typical London street party in 1953 celebrating the coronation of Queen Elizabeth II.

grooves in, with a camera car driving alongside you, and trying to steer it in exactly the same way for several 'takes' and say lines!'

Bicycle ownership was rare for youngsters. Scooters were popular, while go-carts made from pram wheels and orange boxes were a common sight. As a child, I once saw some small boys tie two dogs to a go-cart in an attempt to recreate the chariot from the epic film *Ben Hur*. It made an impressive sight and attracted a cheering crowd – until the dogs charged round a corner and the go-cart collided with a wall.

For all the joy of *Call the Midwife*'s lines of laundry, for all the glory of its swathes of CGI, perhaps the things that most warm the heart about its street scenes are the children. We have hordes of them – jumping, whooping and skirling through the alleyways like vivid diminutive ghosts. They are the children Jenny Lee might have delivered, together with the tireless cycling nuns. Children who grew up and moved out of our sightlines after their homes were razed to rubble, all lost to the light of day.

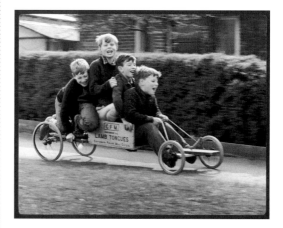

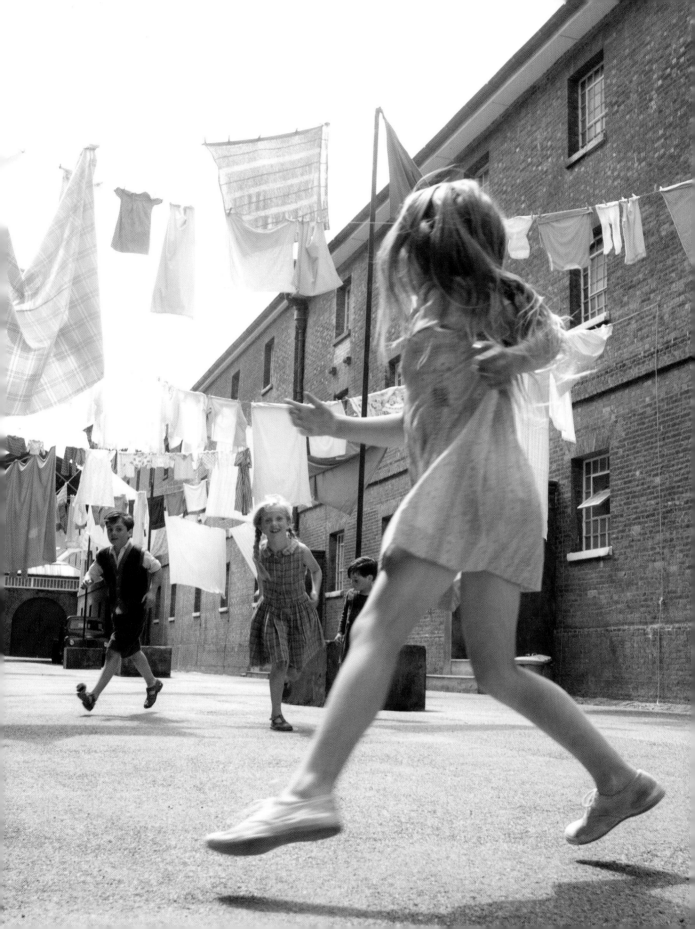

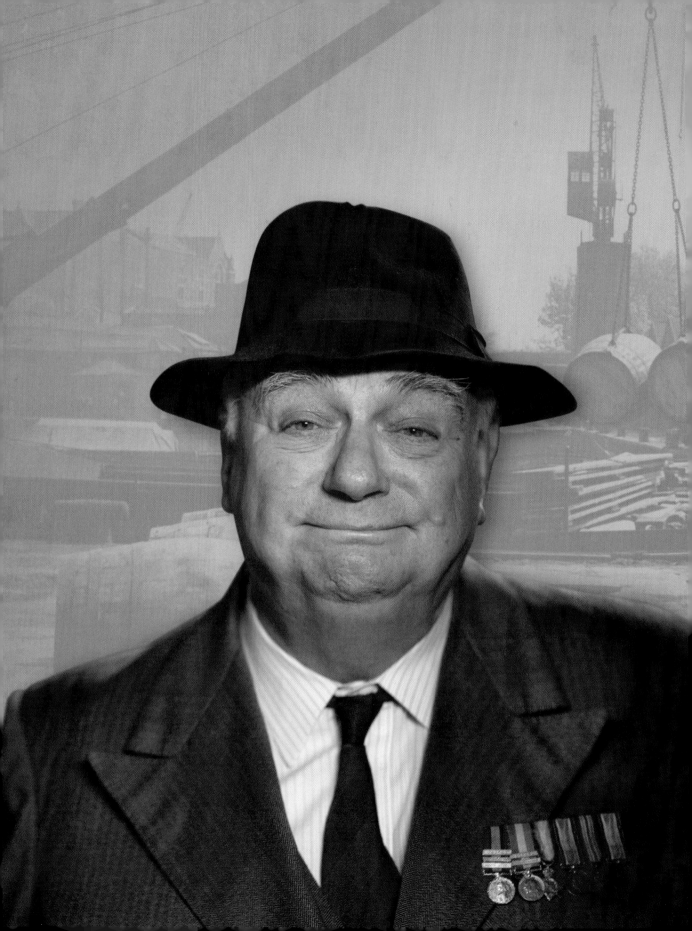

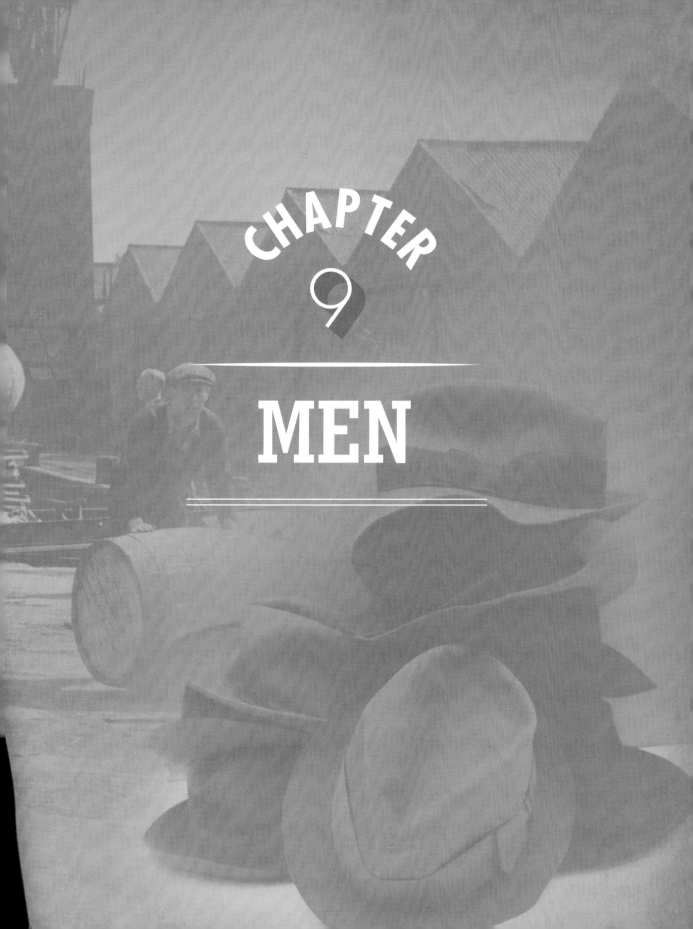

CHAPTER
9

MEN

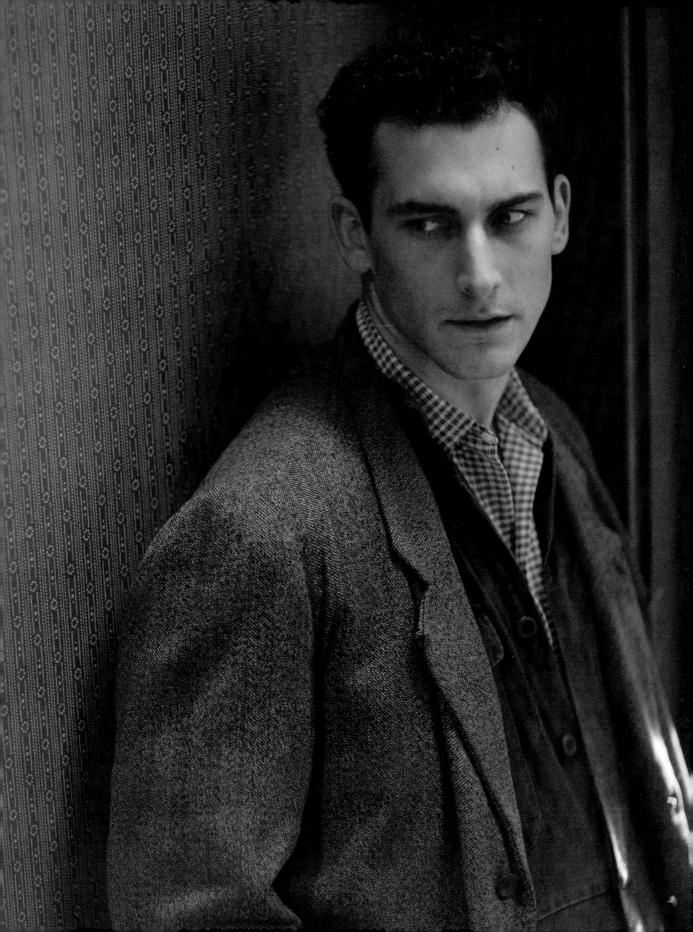

MEN

'NO MAN HAS EVER BEEN ALLOWED
IN ONE OF MY DELIVERY ROOMS, MURIEL.
AND NO MAN EVER SHALL BE.'

SISTER EVANGELINA

When it was suggested to me that this book should include a chapter titled 'Men', my first thought was, 'Well, that'll be quite short.' I then felt rather mean. For all the emphasis on female issues, *Call the Midwife* features some memorable male characters. Who could forget saintly Ted, whose acceptance of his wife's mixed-race baby was so humbling? Or Frank, whose devotion to his sister Peggy broke all moral bounds? Men also play a crucial part behind the scenes. Hugh Warren produces, with Chris Aird as our BBC Executive. And several episodes of Series One were directed, superbly, by Jamie Payne.

Nevertheless, in the world of retro childbirth, the male is a shadowy presence; locked out of delivery rooms, on the margins of the scene. Only Len Warren, veteran father of 25 children, dared to brave convention and stay at his wife's side during labour. He was so expert in matters of childbirth that he could correct Jenny Lee on matters of procedure, and chat with amiable insouciance about Conchita's periods. 'Oh,' he says, breezily, 'She ain't had none of them in years. She's had all the babies one after the other.'

By the standards of the fifties, Len was unusual, if not bordering on freakish, but even he balked at changing nappies. 'Maureen!' he shouted to his teenaged daughter, holding an offending baby at arm's length. 'Come and see to Denise, she needs her drawers changing!'

Children were women's work, and pushing prams was frowned on. Men did not cook and gave washing up a wide berth. Despite the fact that among the working class many wives had part-time jobs, such as cleaning and laundry work, looking after the home was entirely their domain.

Tom Colley, who played Ron Redmond in Episode Four.

Many men living in Poplar worked at the East India Docks. This network of canals and basins had opened in 1803, designed to facilitate imports and exports. The term 'dockworker' embraced several different trades. Lightermen steered the flat-bottomed barges that transported goods from ship to shore. Stevedores loaded cargo, watermen loaded passengers. There were customs officials, crane drivers and troops of

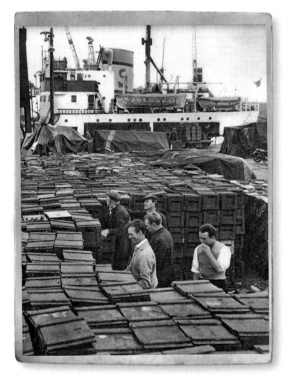

labourers who provided extra hands. The latter group earned a precarious living. Recruitment took place daily, with casual workers gathering outside the dockyard gates – a ritual known as 'The Stand'. Foremen would pick out their favoured workers for a shift, and those overlooked

were left without a wage. Foremen were known to have favourites and immigrant workers were often excluded. Meanwhile, family ties ran deep; membership of a Trades Union could count in your favour – or against.

Politics among dockworkers leant towards the left. A Labour government had followed the World War Two, but this did little to ease industrial relations. When 13,000 dockers went on a strike against wage cuts in 1949, shipping was paralysed for more than three weeks. A London dock strike, with its implications for food imports, had a colossal impact across the capital and the country. Eventually, the Government was forced to send in the army to unload cargo.

There were other sources of employment, in addition to the docks. There was a diesel train maintenance yard at Bow and a ropeworks in Ellesmere Street. Richard Thomas & Baldwins Ltd steelworks was by the dockyard, while wool warehouse Gooch and Cousens did a steady trade. In nearby Silvertown, there was Tate and Lyle Sugar, and in Bow, the Bryant and May Matchworks. Health and safety concerns were virtually unknown, and many people worked in close proximity to toxic gases and asbestos.

Uniformed professions – for those who could get into them – were popular. The dark serge tunics worn by firemen, ambulancemen and prison officers conferred status, and there was the promise of a pension. In *Call the Midwife,* gentle Boer War veteran Joe Collett secures a job for life as a postman. This prevented destitution when old age came to claim him.

Meanwhile, Chummy's beloved, Constable Noakes, has his foot on the first rung of a solid career ladder. Already swotting for Sergeant's exams ('I've been studying the Betting and Gambling Act, the Licensing Act and the

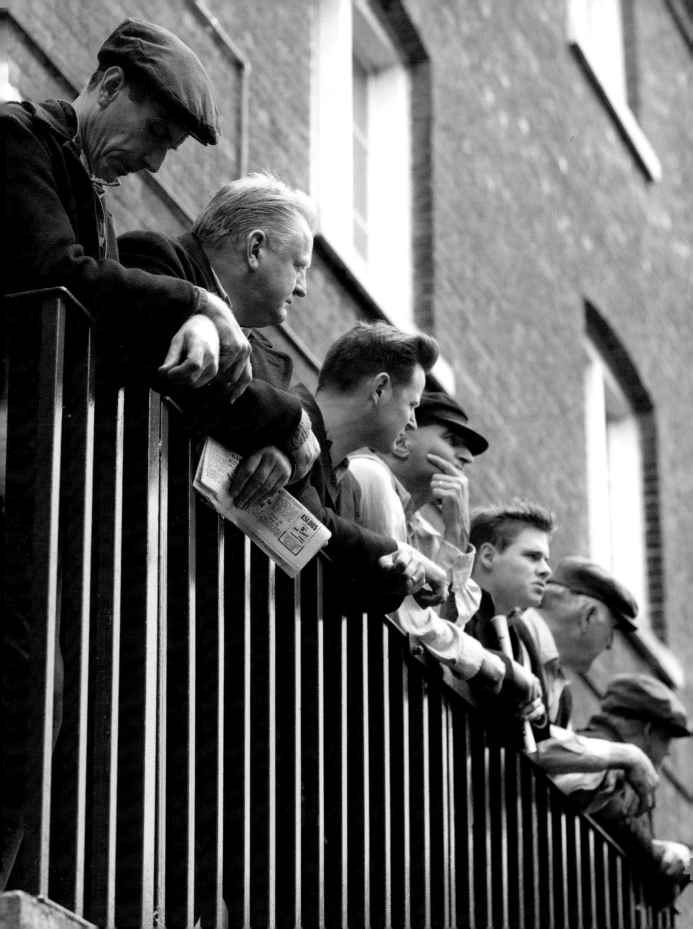

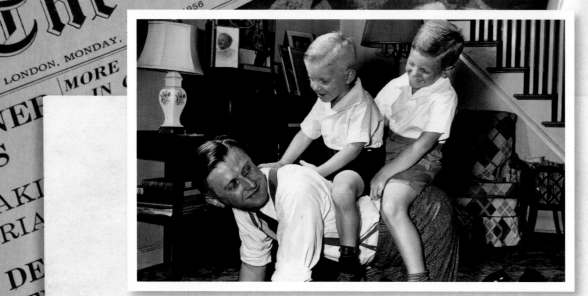

Prostitution Act,' he tells Chummy's unimpressed mother), he can hope to progress to Inspector in due course. Subsidised police housing is the icing on the cake.

Jimmy, Jenny's childhood friend and would-be suitor, is grammar school educated and aspires to a career in architecture. However, in the East End, unless they were extremely bright, most boys left education at 15. If they had been to a technical school, they would hope to be recruited into an apprenticeship in the building trade, or electrical and engineering industries. These earn-as-you-learn training schemes were highly respected, as although it might mean three, five or even seven years on a paltry wage, a boy would enter manhood with that most prized of things – a trade.

Those who did not secure an apprenticeship would be recruited into unskilled jobs in factories, warehouses and offices, doing such menial tasks as sweeping floors or making tea. 'Teaboy' jobs in offices were highly sought after, as they might lead to an opening as a clerk or draughtsman – respectable positions that could mean jobs for life.

Fred, the handyman at Nonnatus House, left school at 14, with little in the way of prospects. A life of manual labour beckoned, but this was not looked upon as a failure in Poplar. It was instead revered as good honest toil – few would choose a life of unremitting, repetitive hard graft, and to embrace and do it well was a badge of honour. After a strenuous war spent digging Other Ranks latrines near El Alamein, Fred decided to put this badge of honour to one side. Having secured a semi-casual position with the nuns, Fred now has several hours a day to spend on profitable projects. Thus far, these have included breeding quails and pigs, making toffee apples, and the sale of (accidentally) alcoholic ginger beer.

The ability to earn a wage and support a family was vital. Marriages happened quite early, a rite of passage in a world that liked tradition and coherence. Courtship was an odd mixture of the rowdy and the formal, centred on dancing and the cinema. Sex – if indulged in at all – was fraught with the danger of conception. If a girl became pregnant, you married her, whether love came into the picture or not.

Whatever the state of play at the altar, children tended to appear within a year or so of marriage. Unless the story specifically states otherwise, we make a point when casting *Call the Midwife* of choosing very young actors to play the babies' fathers. In Series One, the youthful faces of Ron, Cliff and Eddy – firmly shoved out of the birthing room – are almost haunting, and entirely right for the fifties. No matter how welcome the baby, it meant the expense of an extra mouth to feed, and the loss of the mother's wage. Most working-class girls had a job in their teens, perhaps in a shop or a factory, but once they were pregnant they were obliged to leave.

It was often a fight to make ends meet. In working-class homes a cash economy usually operated, with the weekly wage (if the man was in steady employment) brought home in a small brown envelope. Men generally handed their wives an allowance, to cover rent, fuel, clothing and food for the family. The rest was theirs, to spend as they desired.

In the workplace there was very occasionally a cheering glimpse of sexism reversed. Nursing was seen as a female domain and several teaching hospitals refused to take male students until the 1960s. There were, nevertheless, rewards for the brave who made it through. Antonia Bruce, who inspired the character of Trixie in the *Call the Midwife* books, showed me a snap of her graduating class at nursing school. One lone man loomed among the twenty seated girls. Antonia revealed that she and her fellow females had been incensed when they discovered he was paid more than them for doing identical work.

However, the defining facet of the post-War male experience was something from which women were utterly excused. From 1947, the British government operated a peacetime conscription programme for young males, known as National Service. Call-up came at the age of 18, and all who passed the medical served in the army, navy or air force for two years. There was certainly plenty for Jimmy and his peers to do – 100,000 men were needed to occupy Germany, and from 1950 to 1953 there was a war in Korea. British troops were deployed in territories as diverse and faraway as Kenya, Hong Kong, Cyprus and Palestine. For the 6,000 men recruited every fortnight, National Service changed their lives.

Education and apprenticeships were disrupted, budding romances put on hold, and there was an ever-present risk of injury or death.

Some conscripts thrived and many learned new skills, but for others National Service was a torment. In an almost entirely male environment, they were subject to daily drill and hours of 'bulling' kit. Upon discharge they were turned out into the world with a free 'demob' suit and offered – as a last hurrah – total extraction of their teeth and some complimentary dentures.

> *Every National Service graduate knew how to bull his boots and this skill remained conspicuous in Civvy Street.*

Should we wonder then, that fifties' men were sometimes authoritarian, or that they had trouble expressing their emotions? That women frightened them a bit, or that they struggled to cook for themselves? It wasn't all gloom, as they all knew how to iron, and quite a few sailors learned to knit. Men who had been in the navy – accustomed to cramped space on board ship – were also inclined to be extremely tidy.

It's the shoes that I remember. Every National Service graduate knew how to bull his boots and this skill remained conspicuous in Civvy Street. Even men who worked in hobnails had a pair of Sunday shoes, which would appear on high days and holidays, buffed to a patent shine. A man's shoes said everything about him and, above all else, they spoke of self-respect. This was a mantra they passed on to their children.

My own father took a firm line with his offspring when it came to footwear. Several

nights a week, we sat on the kitchen step cleaning our school shoes under his jaunty supervision. I can still smell the cake of Cherry Blossom polish and hear the scuff of the softly bristled brush.

By the time it was abolished in 1960, for good or for ill, the National Service had made its mark on a generation of young males. Other changes would beset them as the century advanced: women would soon take charge of their own destinies, nudging their husbands to budge up and make room. Men saw their world shift as Britain's industrial might first dwindled, then died. The London docks, which had sustained the East End for generations, finally closed when the twisting Thames could not accommodate the vast container ships that now ruled freight. The East India Docks hung on until 1967, when they were razed or filled in, and built over. Today, the wind whistles down the river and around the plate glass columns of the new commercial district. But the young men of the fifties are still with us, if hard work, asbestos or National Service did not kill them. The lovers and the fighters are now grey-haired, and perhaps a little stooped, but they're game for pushing their great-grandchildren's prams, and might even change a nappy if the chips are down. And, on special occasions, they polish their shoes.

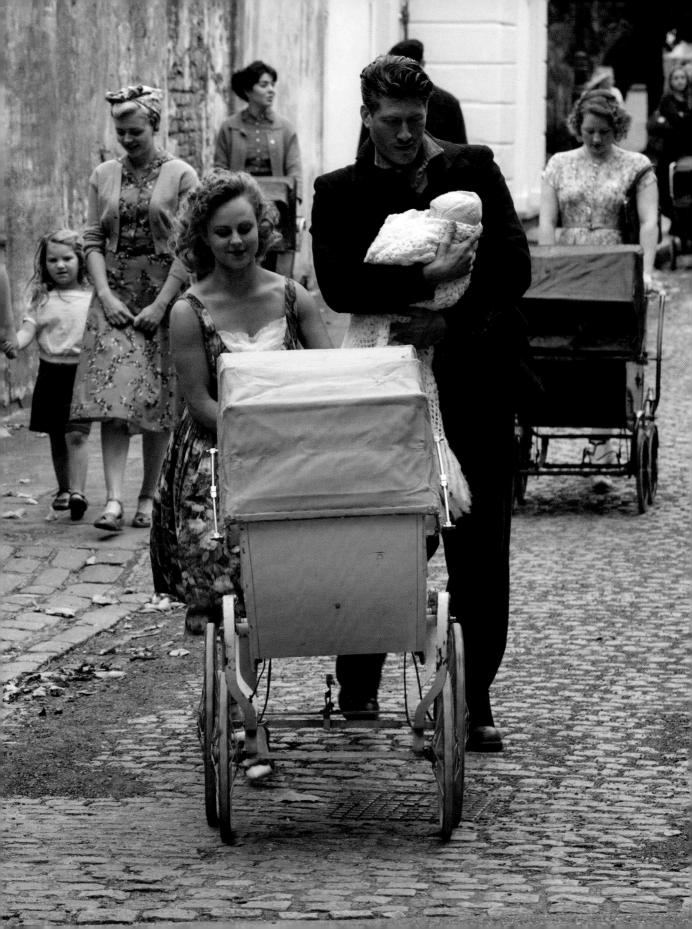

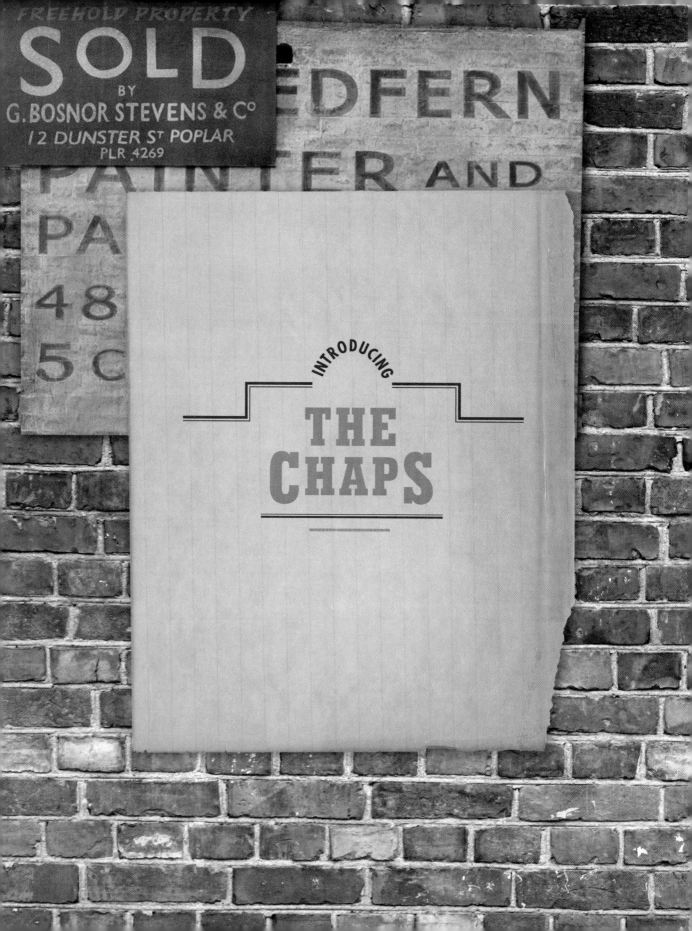

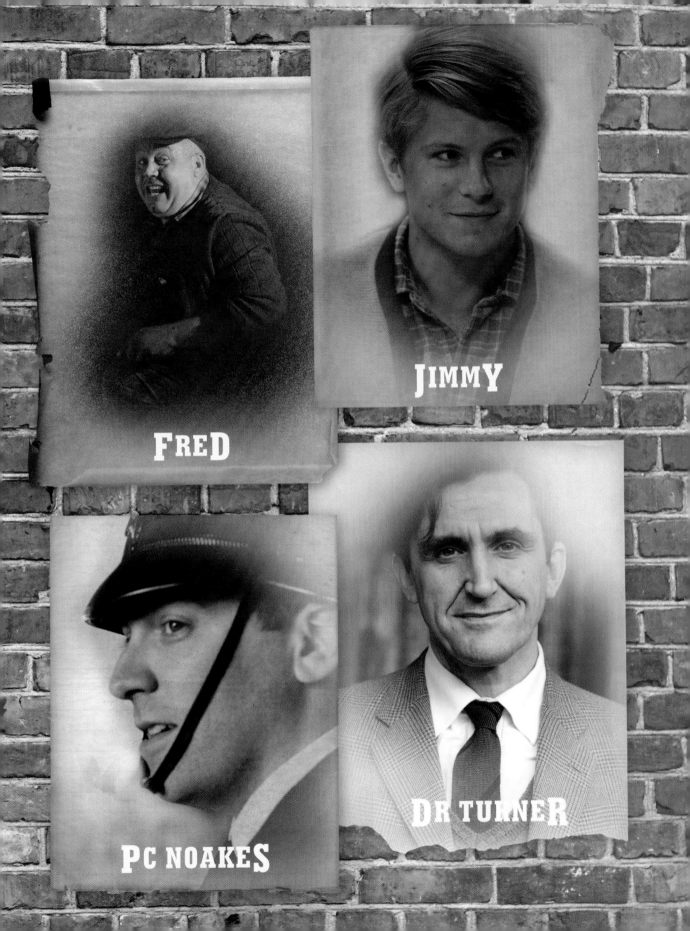

FRED

JIMMY

PC NOAKES

DR TURNER

PROFILE

FRED

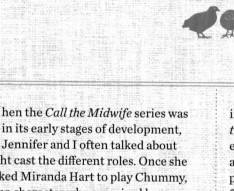

When the *Call the Midwife* series was in its early stages of development, Jennifer and I often talked about how we might cast the different roles. Once she had earmarked Miranda Hart to play Chummy, there was one character who exercised her more than any other – and that was Fred, the convent handyman. In her books he had bowed legs, a spectacular squint and one tooth only. I privately doubted that such a specimen existed, and if he did, whether he was likely to be engaged in the acting profession. I knew within moments of watching Cliff Parisi's audition tape, however, that he would be perfect. His performance had warmth, humour and just the right amount of pomposity and, he was a genuine East Ender. We decided to overlook his healthy set of gnashers.

Cliff embraced the character of Fred, and immediately made him his own. He also revelled in the fact that the tough, emotional tales of *Call the Midwife* were set on his home turf. But his empathy for the material deepened still further after his mother Irene revealed details of his own personal story, which she had kept under wraps for half a century.

Irene fell pregnant with Cliff's older sister when she was just 16, and set up home with the baby's teenaged father in a rented flat in Hackney. There was an acute housing shortage in the late 1950s, and they were lucky to find anywhere at all. However, Cliff was conceived shortly after his sister's birth, and the landlady responded to this second pregnancy in a rather startling way.

'She couldn't have children herself, and she told Mum and Dad they couldn't stay unless they gave her the child. So they had to do a deal with her to just stay in their accommodation,' explained Cliff, who was born in May 1960.

'Obviously, when my mum came back from hospital with me she wouldn't give me or my sister up. So the landlady threw us all out.' The housing crisis in the East End compounded their woes.

'My parents came from big families, but they were all cramped up in one room. No one physically had the space for them, or they would have taken them in.'

Cliff spent his first nights on earth sleeping rough in Victoria Park. Soon afterwards, 'the Welfare' got wind of the family's plight, and arrived at the park to take custody of the children. Cliff's parents – still only 17 and 18 years old – were terrified.

'Mum and Dad jumped on a bus with us, but it was chased by a police car and stopped. Me and my sister were ripped from their arms, and they were left sobbing at the side of the road.'

Both Cliff and his sister were put into care in Reading, too far distant for their parents to visit. However, George and Irene both found jobs, and worked tirelessly towards reclaiming their children. Once they had secured the Holy Grail of rented accommodation, the family was reunited.

'When my mum told me that story last year, I was quite upset. I didn't know who I felt more sorry for, them or me. It was a bit shocking.'

Cliff went on to enjoy a carefree childhood playing out on the streets of Hornsey, North London, where his parents settled. Academically Cliff didn't shine at school. 'I was dyslexic, but in those days you were just labelled thick.' He left school at the age of 13 with a passionate desire to act, but it was impossible to get into drama school without academic qualifications. By the mid-1980s, Cliff had become a successful stand-up comic, which earned him an Equity card. A fully paid-up member of the performers' union, he was finally able to turn his hand to acting.

Warmth and humour are at the forefront of Cliff's performance as Fred. However, Cliff is conscious there's a different side to the handyman's life. 'Fred lost his wife and several of his children in the Blitz. Now, he sees the nuns and the girls as his family. They are pretty much all he has got. At the same time, he sees opportunities to make a few quid presenting themselves. He is still looking to make his fortune. He hasn't given up on life at all.'

Asked if there's a downside to playing Fred, Cliff responds without hesitation – it is the distinctive moustache that he himself suggested. 'I hate it,' he says. 'So does the wife.'

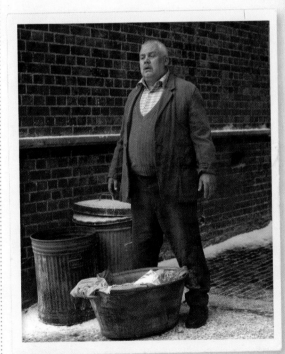

Q&A

What's your favourite item of clothing?
Denim overalls. I bought three sets down the Army and Navy – one on, one off, one in the wash. And any stubborn stains, you can set to with the Vim.

Where do you go on holiday?
I'm not especially partial to sleeping in strange beds. A charabanc outing does me nicely, especially if it's headed for somewhere with a pier. When I'm looking at the sea I want something solid underneath my feet, not sand. I saw enough sand at El Alamein.

Given the choice, where would you spend Saturday nights?
I should be very sorry to see the Pig and Whistle forced out of business due to lack of diligence from its clientele. So I'd go down there, and demonstrate my support for an historic hostelry.

What do you do in your spare time?
I came to the end of the road with fireworks manufacture, and so I swapped the last of the gunpowder for a jigsaw machine. A man must acquire new skills, or die. I'll be carrying on with my series of 300-piece cottage scenes as soon as I get this bandage off my thumb.

What is your favourite meal?
My daughter Dolly makes a prizewinning steak and kidney pudding. She boils it all up in a tea towel, so you can see the creases in the suet. Lovely.

What's your secret vice?
Patience Strong puts a lump in my throat from time to time. I sometimes cut her poems out and put them in my pocket.

And your best quality?
I am unrivalled with a blockage. Sinks. Drains. Khazis. I've even advised on bowels, though only within the family circle.

What's your most treasured memory?
VE Day. I kissed a WAAF I'd never met, just off Piccadilly Circus, then caught the bus and came straight home to Poplar, duty done.

If you had a motto, what would it be?
Hard work never killed anyone. But it has put a few backs out.

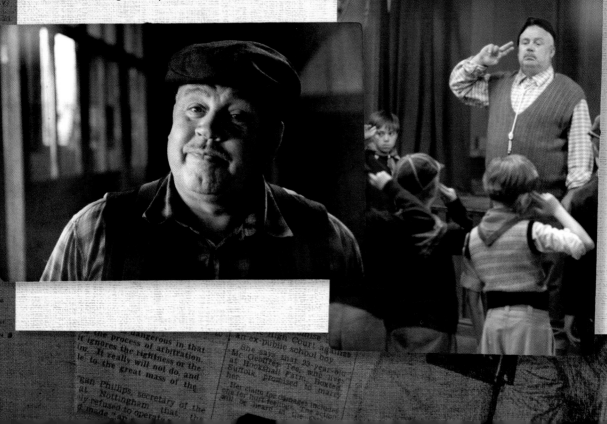

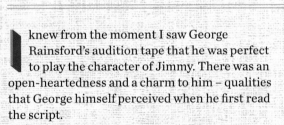

PROFILE

JIMMY

I knew from the moment I saw George Rainsford's audition tape that he was perfect to play the character of Jimmy. There was an open-heartedness and a charm to him – qualities that George himself perceived when he first read the script.

'I really liked that Jimmy came without any dark baggage. He was a genuinely nice, expansive sort of guy. But he's also optimistic and romantic, and it leaves him open to being hurt – later on, that becomes quite interesting to play.'

George was born in Huddersfield and educated at Repton in Derbyshire, where his mother taught French. School plays fired an early love of drama, but it was appearing at the Edinburgh Fringe that sealed his wish to act. 'I played Mozart in Peter Schaffer's *Amadeus*, and the whole role was just amazing.'

After finishing a drama degree at the University of Manchester, George committed to professional training at the London Academy of Music and Dramatic Art. Television parts in *Doctors*, *Law and Order* and *Waking the Dead* followed, along with plays at the Royal Court and National Theatres and with the RSC. George jumped at the chance to work with Jessica Raine in *Call the Midwife*. 'We already knew each other socially, and we laugh together very easily. Jimmy and Jenny have known each other for years, and it was great just to use that rapport.'

He is less enamoured of Jimmy's 1950s' haircut. Married in the summer of 2012, he reports that his new wife, actress Jaimi Barbakoff, thinks it makes him look like a 'choir boy'.

George says his most memorable day on set came when shooting Episode Four of Series One. In glorious sunshine, Jimmy, Jenny and a host

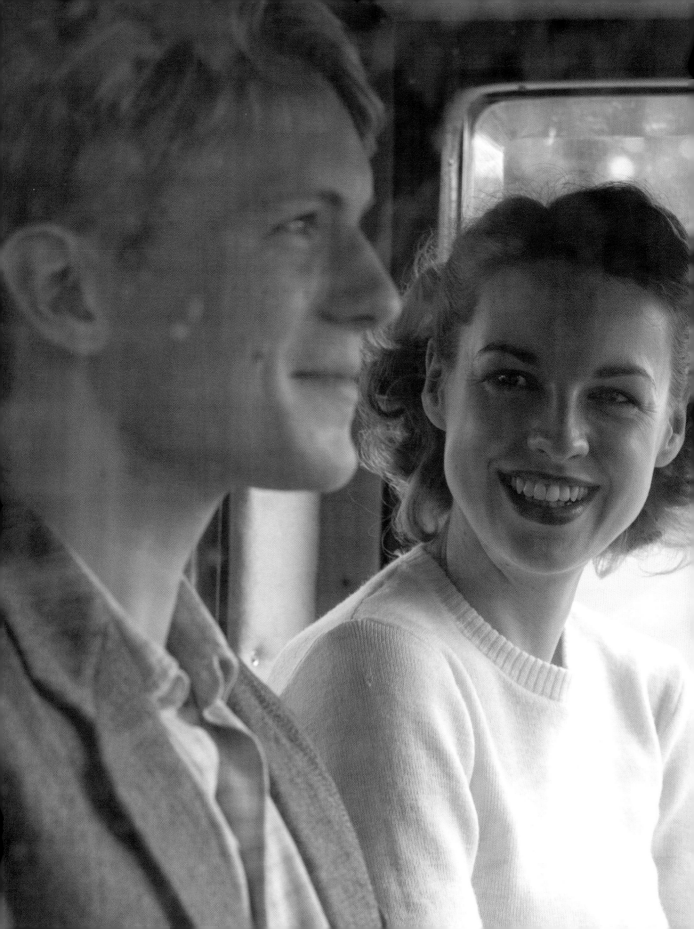

of friends visited an abandoned country house in Jimmy's car. At that point, George did not have a driver's licence. 'I had only had three lessons in my life, but we were on private land, so they put me behind the wheel.' Confronted with grinding vintage gears, George was already nervous. 'Then they told me the car was worth about £80,000. Then they fixed a camera to the side of it, and somebody said it was worth £250,000. Then the three leading ladies of the show got in the back – and they told me to drive towards the house at thirty miles an hour.' George admits to being terrified, but adds, 'Between Series One and Series Two, I made sure I passed my test!'

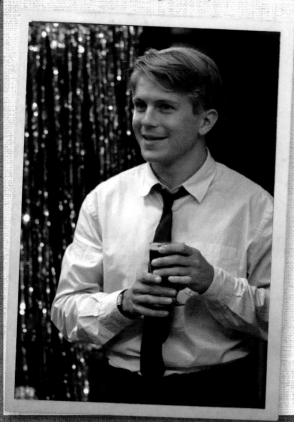

Q&A

What's your favourite item of clothing?
My demob suit. I was given it on my last day of National Service and I've never loved any garment as much before or since.

Where do you go on holiday?
I'm hatching a plan to drive Lady Chatterley, my converted hearse, as far as Spain. I was hoping that if we drive via Paris, Jenny might be persuaded to come with me.

Given the choice, where would you spend Saturday nights?
Somewhere different every week. But there must be beer.

What do you do in your spare time?
I'm swotting for architect's exams, and I'm also teaching myself to play the double bass. I've wanted to learn ever since I went to Ronnie Scott's jazz club.

What is your favourite meal?
A Melton Mowbray pork pie, while I'm driving.

What's your secret vice?
I'd go slightly too far out of my way to look at a photograph of Princess Margaret.

And your best quality?
When I fix my heart on something, I will not let it go.

What's your most treasured memory?
It's somebody's face. And she is laughing.

If you had a motto, what would it be?
Hold fast to that which is good.

PROFILE
PC NOAKES

When PC Noakes married his beloved Chummy – or Camilla, as he calls her – there were two special guests in the crowd. As the happy couple emerged from church, his wife Emma and three-month-old son Bertie were among the extras standing on the steps.

'Look Bertie!' Emma whispered in the baby's ear. 'There's Daddy ... and he's getting married.'

For actor Ben Caplan, taking your son to work is one of the perks of working on *Call the Midwife*. He admits he has been 'blown away' by the arrival of his child. 'Just watching him develop and grow, I cannot tell you how amazing it has been.'

Ben admits to weeping when he saw a re-run of Episode Two of *Call the Midwife* in which Chummy took charge in a difficult breech birth. 'I was there throughout Emma's 36-hour labour, so I appreciate that this show doesn't shy away from the realities of childbirth.'

The way Ben sees it, PC Noakes is one of the good guys. 'There's a real sense of chivalry about him, he's very straight but always very respectful. I really warm to him as a character.'

The pivotal relationship between himself and Chummy, played by comedienne Miranda Hart, fell into place at once.

'They come together because there are similarities between them. Neither is particularly comfortable in their own skin. We had a rehearsal before we started filming and it felt very easy. And Miranda and I got on well together when we were just hanging out. I identified with him, and I think she identified with Chummy. I love PC Noakes' simplicity – he loves Chummy for who she is, and he's not worried by appearances. She is very authentic.'

For Ben, the extraordinary response to the series was something of a surprise. 'We always knew there was a lot about this show, and we hoped people would take to it, but I don't think we ever had a sense of what it would become. The scripts are so beautifully written, the characters are so affectionately created, and I think that is what is attracting people.'

Success has yet to change Ben's life. He has also appeared in *Band of Brothers*, *A Touch of Frost* and *Judge John Deed* on television. But post-*Call the Midwife*, PC Noakes' comb-over hair, policeman's cape and specs have been sufficient to preserve his anonymity.

'I went on holiday earlier this year and across the aisle of the plane a woman was reading the book. She didn't recognise me. I thought about leaning over and asking what she thought of the television show, but in the end I didn't risk it.'

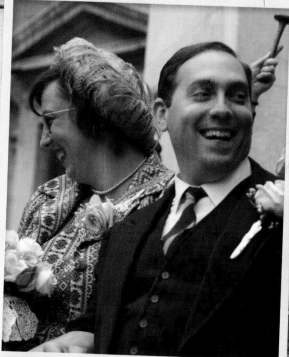

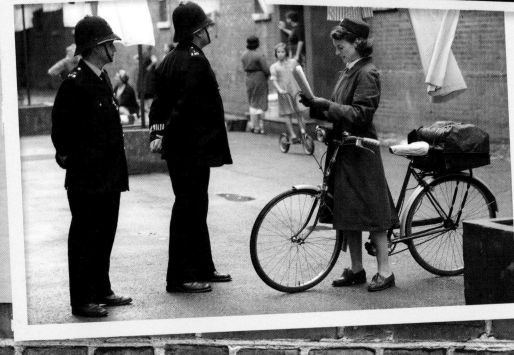

Q&A

What's your favourite item of clothing?
Until I got married, I would have said my uniform. Now, I would say my slippers. I'm never happier than when I'm at home with my wife.

Where do you go on holiday?
We went to Ramsgate for our honeymoon. But when I was a nipper, I used to go to my uncle's farm in Kent.

Given the choice, where would you spend Saturday nights?
At the pictures. I like a good Western, but Camilla goes in for musicals. Trouble is, she thinks I do too because I told a white lie on our first date, and I've never had the heart to tell her I was fibbing. *Gigi* this weekend, and it serves me right.

What do you do in your spare time?
We're on the waiting list for an allotment. I like the feeling of soil on my hands, it goes back to helping dig potatoes on the farm.

What is your favourite meal?
My dad's cousin was a waiter at a kosher restaurant called Bloom's. We used to go and see him there, and he'd bring us bowls of chicken soup with knedlach, which are the best dumplings you've ever tasted.

What's your secret vice?
The Beano.

And your best quality?
I can calm people down when they panic. Even when I'm panicking inside.

What's your most treasured memory?
Waking up in a boarding house in Ramsgate and seeing Camilla's wedding hat lying on the floor.

If you had a motto, what would it be?
God loves a trier.

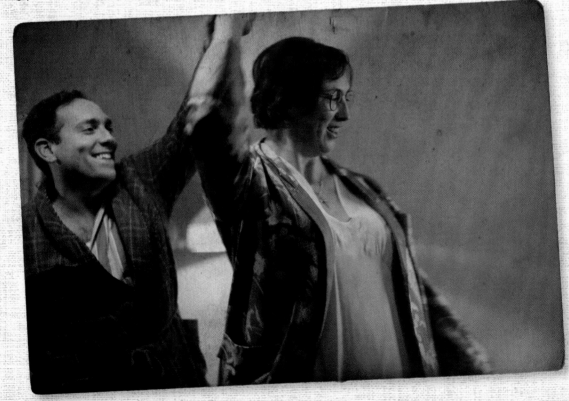

PROFILE

DR TURNER

Perhaps uniquely among the cast of the series, Stephen McGann (who happens to be my husband) was delivered by a midwife who arrived by bike. 'I was born during a blizzard in the freezing cold winter of 1963,' he reveals. 'The midwife left her bike outside when she arrived soon after midnight. My mother endured a long labour, and next morning the bike had to be dug out of the snow.'

Stephen suffered chest problems as a child, and enjoyed an early taste of the limelight when he was taken to hospital by ambulance suffering from pneumonia. 'I can remember a small crowd gathering in the street to see me being stretchered into the ambulance,' he says. 'And I made sure I looked especially poorly for my audience.'

His early experiences have given him a keen appreciation of the value of free health care, and he jumped at the chance to audition for the role of Dr Turner.

'He is a deeply good man. He is a vocational doctor who works desperately hard. He is always tired. He works incessantly for the people on his watch,' says Stephen. 'However, he's also a man of his time. In the 1950s, nurses had to defer to the doctor in a way they don't quite so much now. Doctors did have a habit of swanning in and taking all the credit, at the time when the groundwork had been done by women.'

Above all else, Stephen sees *Call the Midwife* as a celebration of the optimism that surrounded the National Health Service. 'It's just an amazing and honourable system,' he remarks, 'in which everyone is essentially sacred. Everybody matters, no matter how poor they are.'

With this in mind, given the choice of two suits by costume designer Amy Roberts, he plumped for

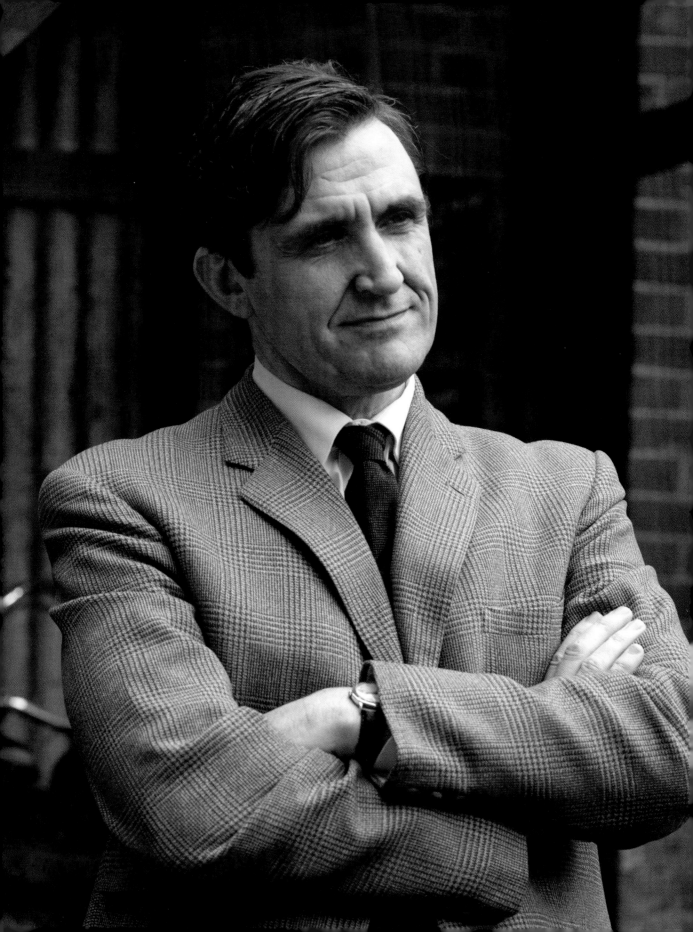

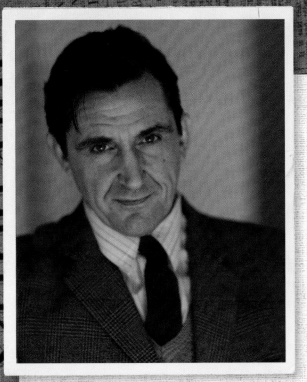

one with a small darn on the knee. 'It seemed to say so much about this dedicated doctor,' he says. 'He works among the poor and isn't that well off himself. He is literally kneeling at his patient's bedsides, wearing himself to a thread in their service.'

Stephen is delighted by *Call the Midwife*'s painstaking attention to detail. 'Everything is so carefully researched, both at the script stage and during filming,' he says. 'For the Christmas episode, I was trained in exactly how to conduct an ear examination using an instrument correct for the period. It is also absolutely right that Dr Turner smokes – at the time, some brands of cigarette were actually endorsed by doctors!'

Stephen takes a keen interest in all things pertaining to the history of science and medicine. He balances his acting career with academic pursuits, and will graduate from Imperial College, London with a Master's degree in Science Communication in the spring of 2013.

Q&A

What's your favourite item of clothing?
I have a scarf that was a gift from my wife a few weeks before she died. I live in dread of losing it.

Where do you go on holiday?
I haven't taken a holiday for three years – it's impossible to find a reliable locum for the practice. But this summer I might manage a weekend's fishing on the River Test.

Given the choice, where would you spend Saturday nights?
At the theatre, watching Shakespeare, or perhaps a farce – I don't mind what I see, as long as it makes me laugh or cry. And in an ideal world, no one in the audience would collapse, and I wouldn't have to resuscitate them in the aisle. It has happened.

What do you do in your spare time?
I spend it all with my son, Timothy.

What is your favourite meal?
A full English breakfast, though not necessarily at breakfast time. The East End is full of little cafés, and when I'm on my rounds I'm never very far from a plateful of bacon, eggs, tomatoes, sausage and fried bread.

What's your secret vice?
Extra fried bread.

And your best quality?
I've learned how to listen.

What's your most treasured memory?
The queue of people outside my surgery on 5 July 1948, the day the National Health was born.

If you had a motto, what would it be?
'Treat often, cure sometimes, comfort always.'

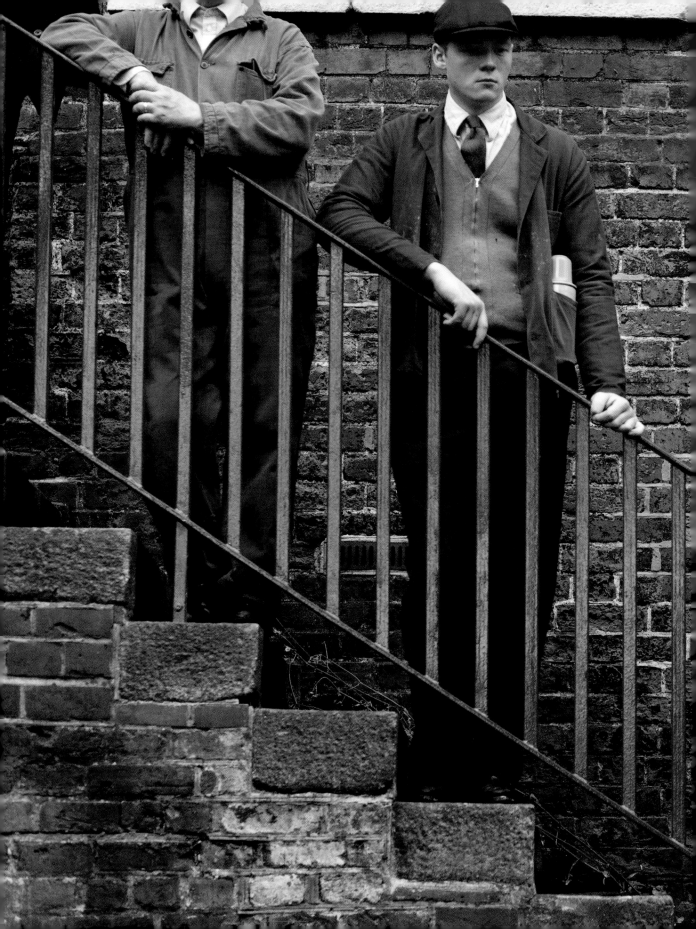

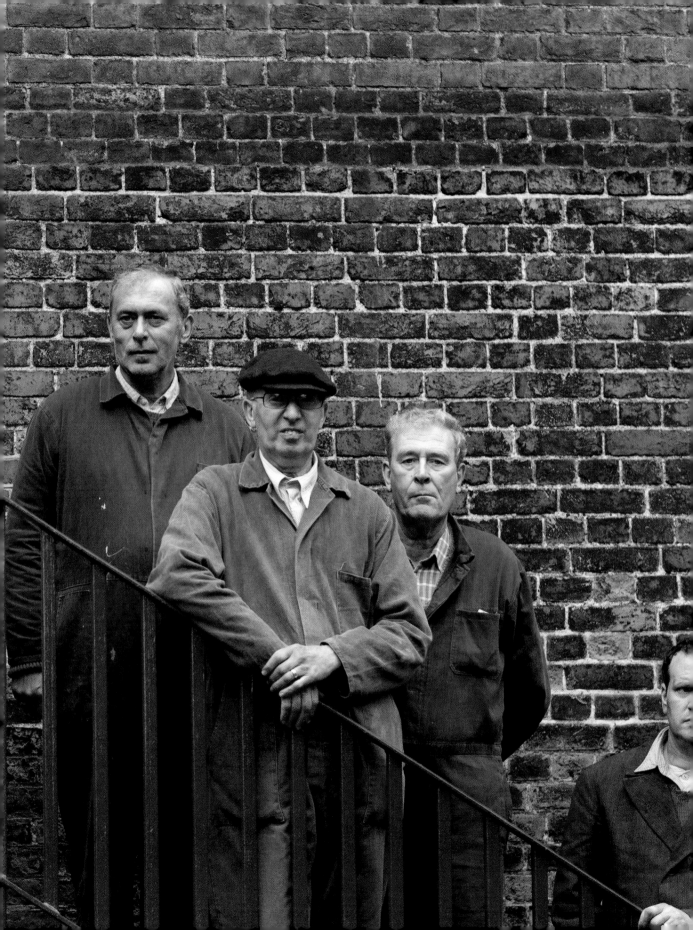

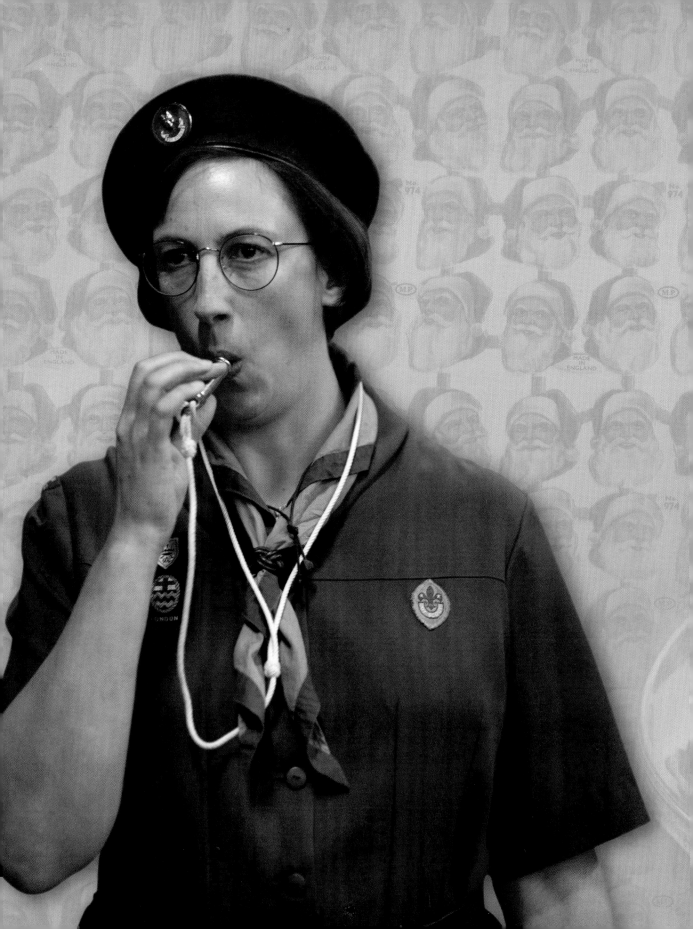

CHAPTER
10

CHRISTMAS

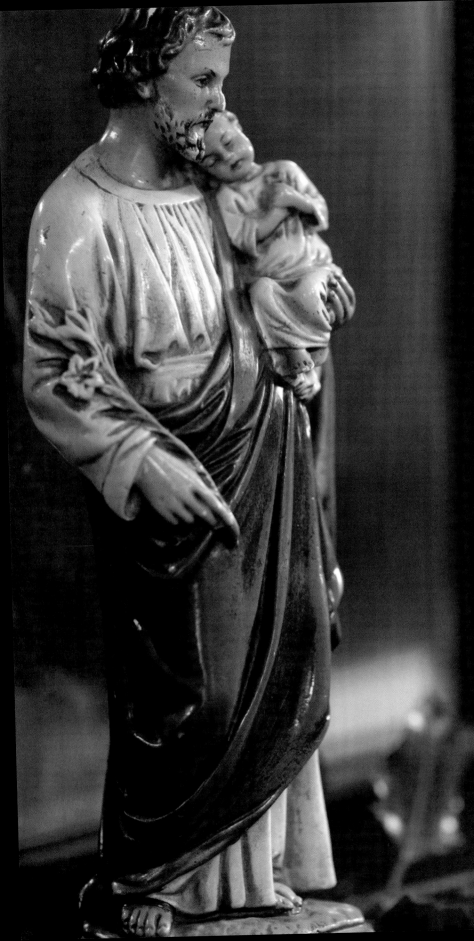

CHRISTMAS

'YOU WON'T BE LAUGHING COME THE CUBS'
NATIVITY. HOW WILL IT LOOK LIKE BETHLEHEM,
WITHOUT A TREE, AND LIGHTS?'
FRED

When we were first invited to make a Christmas episode of *Call the Midwife*, we hesitated – for about five minutes. Yes, it would be challenging to recreate a wintry Poplar during a July shoot, but as Pippa Harris said, 'Christmas is *about* the birth of a baby. Above all else, it celebrates the arrival of new life, and that is the very essence of this show.'

The prospect, in the end, proved irresistible. By high summer, Chummy – in her new role as Akela – was directing the Cubs' nativity play, and the steps of Nonnatus House shone white with snow.

The tinsel and the lights of a fifties' Christmas look similar, at first glance, to those we relish in the present day. But there are differences, and they say much about the journey we have been on in the meantime.

The festive episode of *Call the Midwife* opens with Sister Julienne praying in the chapel; in the kitchen, Jenny Lee scrubs the Nativity set, leaving the shepherds to dry on the draining board. In religious communities, preparation still begins with Advent, a period of prayer and reflection that starts on 1 December. But nowadays the shops unveil their decorations in October. Sixty years ago, festive trimmings stayed under wraps until two weeks beforehand. The build-up was shorter, but the pleasure no less intense.

In the fifties, most cities had large department stores, which laid on a Christmas Grotto experience for children. A magic tunnel lined with pictures or puppet tableaux would lead to an audience with Santa Claus himself, and the chance to choose a toy from a bran tub. For an extra fee, he would pose for a photograph. This foray into commercialism gathered steam across the sixties and seventies, then fizzled out in all

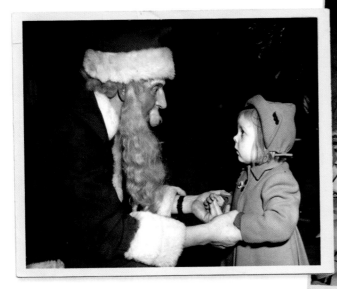

but a handful of venues. Perhaps they failed to thrill a more sophisticated generation.

Christmas was increasingly focused on children's enjoyment. In 1957, Santa's gifts to children were more abundant and expensive than ever before. Meccano, with its red and pea green metal pieces, had been a popular construction toy since the beginning of the century. Meccano also manufactured model cars – the 'Dinky' range – at their premises in Liverpool and these were much desired by small boys. However, in the East End, local pride might have led to 'Matchbox' being the brand of choice. Die-cast Matchbox cars were made by Lesney at their works in Edmonton and sent to the Speigelstein factory in Hackney Wick for metal plating.

A girl might long for a doll called Peach Blossom, sold by Marks & Spencer's for the colossal sum – in the fifties – of 35 shillings. Very much a damsel of the modern age, Peach Blossom was made of vinyl and proudly dressed in nylon. A doughty product of British craftsmanship, she was also guaranteed unbreakable.

In addition there were annuals including *Rupert the Bear* and *Girls' Own*, hula hoops to swing those hips, Muffin the Mule puppets, painting by numbers sets, *I-Spy* books, a yoyo ... And, if parents were practically minded, such dismal treats as new pants or a toothbrush. It was traditional for Father Christmas to leave a tangerine and a few Brazil nuts at the bottom of each stocking. I hope mine was not the only family where the kids were told to put them straight back in the fruit bowl, because they were only for show.

Decorations around the home were simple and sometimes made by hand. Paper chains were popular, fashioned by children from scraps or from packets of ready-pasted paper strips,

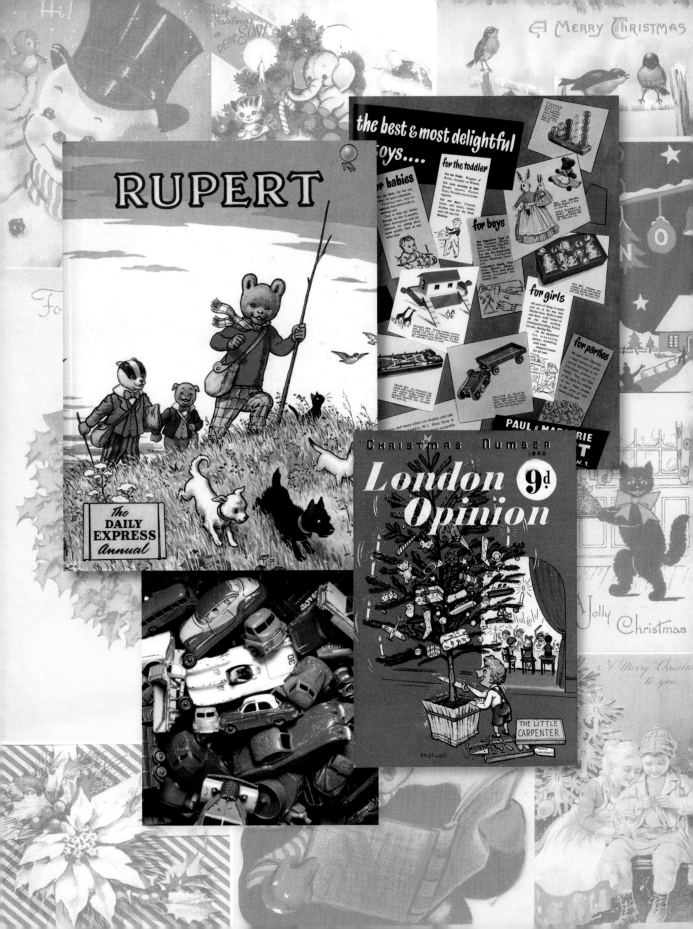

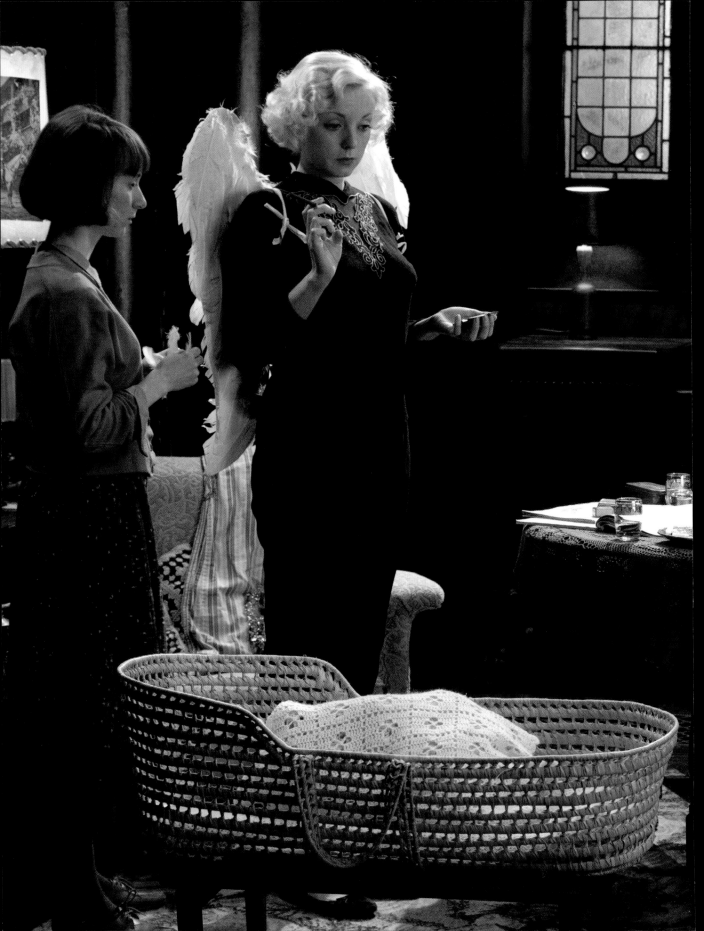

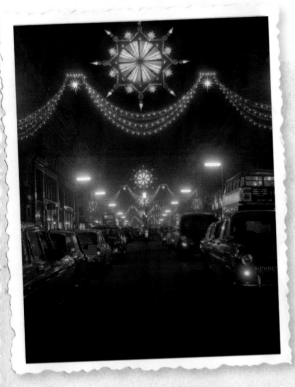

available for pennies at the newsagent. Streamers of crêpe paper trailed from central light fittings to the picture rails. Bells were a popular motif – on Christmas cards or as ornaments. Now we are more likely to decorate with stars.

During World War Two, the cutting down of real Christmas trees was banned and there was a rush to re-embrace the tradition after hostilities ceased. In *Call the Midwife*, Fred takes great pride in putting up a huge spruce in the parish hall.

Many people still decorated their trees with wax candles firmly fixed to thick branches. These were a significant fire hazard, which may explain why trees were not put up and decorated until a week or less before Christmas – if they dried out for too long in the sitting room, a conflagration might ensue. Poignantly, some families clung to the rudimentary 'goose-feather' artificial trees that were standard in the war years. Little more than a stick with a few splayed branches, they

were made up to 18 inches high and designed for tabletop use. But despite their lack of opulence, like all Christmas decorations they became deeply loved, a symbol of all that family meant. My grandparents were still using their tiny wartime tree in the seventies. It was so rickety and bald they took to concealing its defects by hanging it with Mars Bars and packets of Maltesers, which we heartless children thought a great improvement.

As Fred's parish hall tree demonstrates, tinsel came in short, wiry lengths and was made from aluminium or even lead foil. Fairy lights, when used, were basic bulbs of thick primary-coloured glass, linked by a gnarled brown fabric flex, and lasted for years. In contrast to today's Las Vegas style displays, one string per household was the rule. Every December from 1954 onwards, there was a display of Christmas illuminations in London's Regent Street, and Oxford Street followed suit five years later. A trip to 'see the lights' became an annual treat for many East End children – all for the price of a ticket on the 23 bus, which went direct from Poplar to the heart of the shopping district. Front-row, top-deck seats were much prized as they offered a peerless view of the spectacle.

Although church going generally had started to slope off, Christmas still had a strongly religious flavour and Nativity plays majored on Bethlehem. We were careful to reflect this with Chummy's Cub Scout production, in which angels are much featured, and 'Silent Night' is bawled lustily by all. Carol services were common and church attendance on the morning of the 25th was hearty. Midnight Mass was less popular. This is possibly because more people used public transport and didn't fancy walking home in the bus-less Yuletide dark.

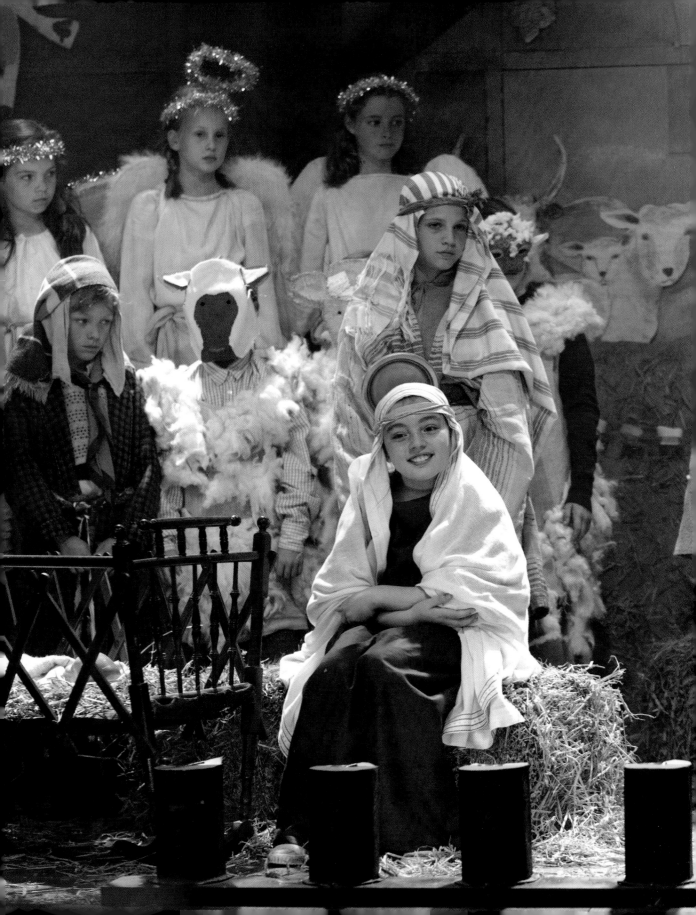

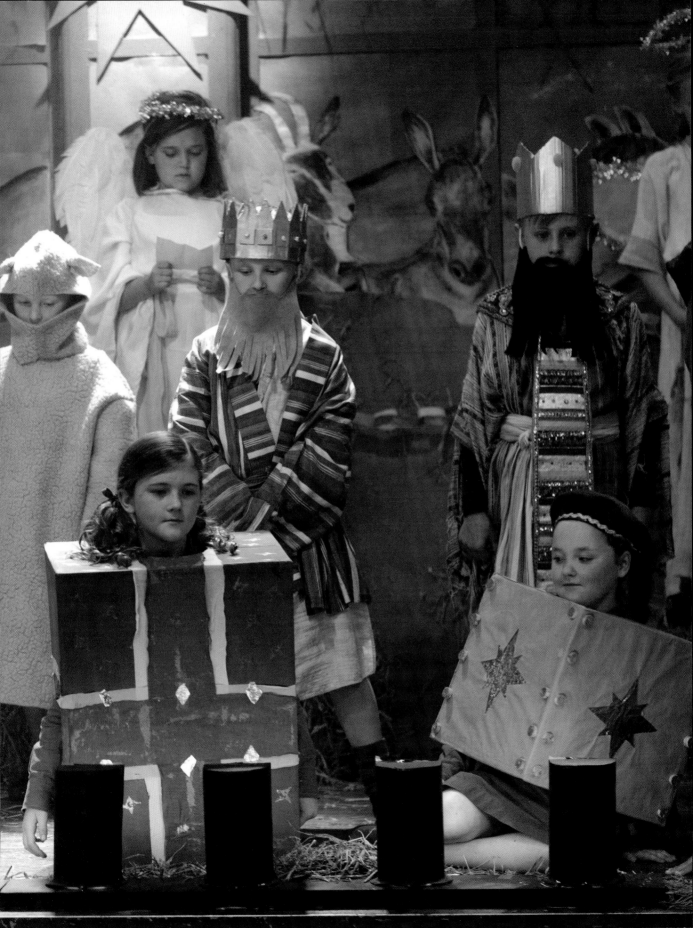

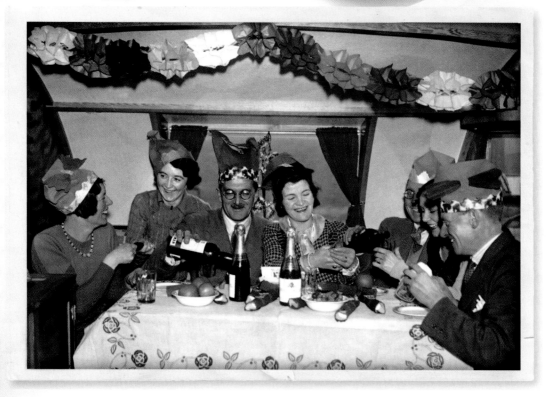

In the fifties, the spirit of a consumer Christmas began to make its presence felt.

A harbinger of this was the sudden emergence of 'Christmas Clubs' – a neat, localised reversal of credit in which housewives banked small weekly sums with specific shopkeepers during the autumn months. Records were kept of the separate sums deposited, and at Christmas the women would visit the grocer, butcher and greengrocer, spending the money put away with something very like abandon.

Specially purchased treats might include pickled walnuts, tinned salmon, soused herrings, glacé fruits and Eat Me dates from France. The fifties also saw the rise of Quality Street, a family treat still essential today. Milk Tray chocolates – 'Every one with a different centre' – appealed to the more sophisticated, and Black Magic to those more sophisticated still. Nothing kept for

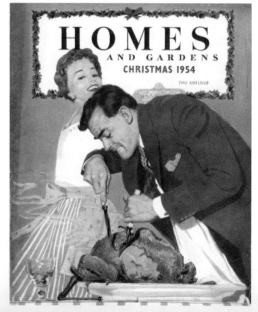

very long in homes that lacked refrigeration, so any cheese course would be modest. It would be accompanied by celery sticks, served standing upright in tumblers full of water.

The centrepiece of Christmas dinner was always almost always a roasted bird. Goose was going out of fashion, but turkey was on the rise, as was the capon – a rooster castrated to improve its flavour. Though large enough to feed an extended family, these were often tough and chicken was preferred. Chicken was kept for high days and holidays in the fifties as there were no intensive farming methods in operation and it cost farmers dearly to fatten up free-range hens. Boxing Day

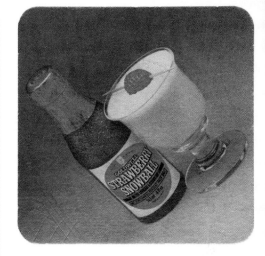

was, as now, a Bank Holiday in Britain and in most homes other than the poorest, another formal sit-down dinner would be served. This would often centre around pork, beef or gammon, alongside cold cuts from the previous day.

The Christmas pudding – if not bought – would have been made as early as September to give the blend of dried fruits and alcohol a good chance to mature. After an initial four-hour steam, it would have been stashed away in a larder or dark cupboard, ready for another three hours' boil on Christmas Eve, and then the same again the following morning. By the time the dinner rolled around, condensation would be sliding down the kitchen walls.

At that time, no one seems to have realised that this dark sticky dessert was not compulsory. If trifle was dished up alongside it – as opposed to being kept until teatime, three hours later – it was intended for any children present. It was considered rather feeble to refuse Christmas pudding, although some got away with just having a mince pie. Both pudding and pies were served with a white cornflour-based sauce, which had

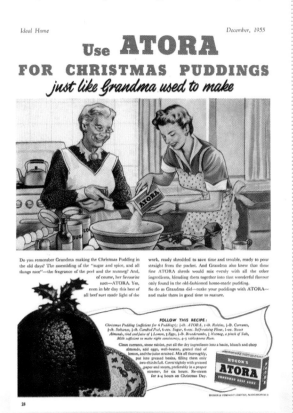

been liberally flavoured with artificial rum or brandy essence. Brandy butter, or 'hard sauce' as it was known to Mrs Beeton, was a costly confection, confined to wealthier homes.

It wouldn't be Christmas without paper hats.

※

Candles on the table seem to be a modern trend. In the fifties, the centrepiece was more likely to be a hollow Santa Claus or snowman containing small novelty gifts. Christmas crackers, a British tradition going back to 1841, were a given. Paper hats have never lost their hold over the British and they, and the crackers they come in, have been transported to every corner of the globe, yet have never caught on in any other culture. We are faintly aware that non-Brits find them risible, but we wear them anyway. It wouldn't be Christmas without paper hats.

In working and even middle-class houses in the fifties, neither wine nor champagne were drunk with Christmas dinner, though there might have been sherry beforehand and a tot of port to follow. In the East End, beer – perhaps a bottled brand such as Watney's Pale Ale – would be brought to the table and drunk from a glass. Babycham, a fizzy drink made from fermented pears, was popular with ladies, as was the 'Snowball', a blend of Warnink's Advocaat (an egg-based Dutch liqueur) and lemonade.

The Christmas cake, like the pudding, would have been made many weeks previously. Not many people were mad on this either, and by New Year most Christmas cakes were reduced to a heap of crumbled rubble on the sideboard. But they remained an essential centrepiece, bound year after year with the same recycled ribbons and topped with robins of brightly painted chalk.

In the evening, board games such as Ludo and Snakes and Ladders might be played, or perhaps – in more middle class homes – the Monopoly would come out. Scrabble had been introduced to the UK in 1955, and was swift to gain in popularity.

In the present day, television is central to our experience of Christmas but in 1957 things were rather different. Most homes had radios and at Christmas, American singer Harry Belafonte was at number 1 in the Hit Parade with 'Mary's Boy Child'.

The new medium of television had been suspended during the War, resuming only in 1946. A 'toddler's truce' had then been imposed by the Government, in which television was blacked out for one hour daily, between 6 and 7pm. This was supposedly so that children could be put to bed believing programmes had finished for the night. This was abandoned in 1957, the same year Pinky and Perky made their debut. The BBC schedule remained very limited, with long periods of the day where only the test card and music were available.

But the cultural impact of the small screen was in the ascendant. On Christmas Day 1957, the Queen addressed the nation on television for the first time. A mere 25 years earlier, her grandfather, King George V, had made his inaugural radio broadcast. Now, two coronations and a World War later, the Royals were breaking new ground once again.

The clip, seen now, makes for touching viewing. Her Majesty faces the camera at a slight

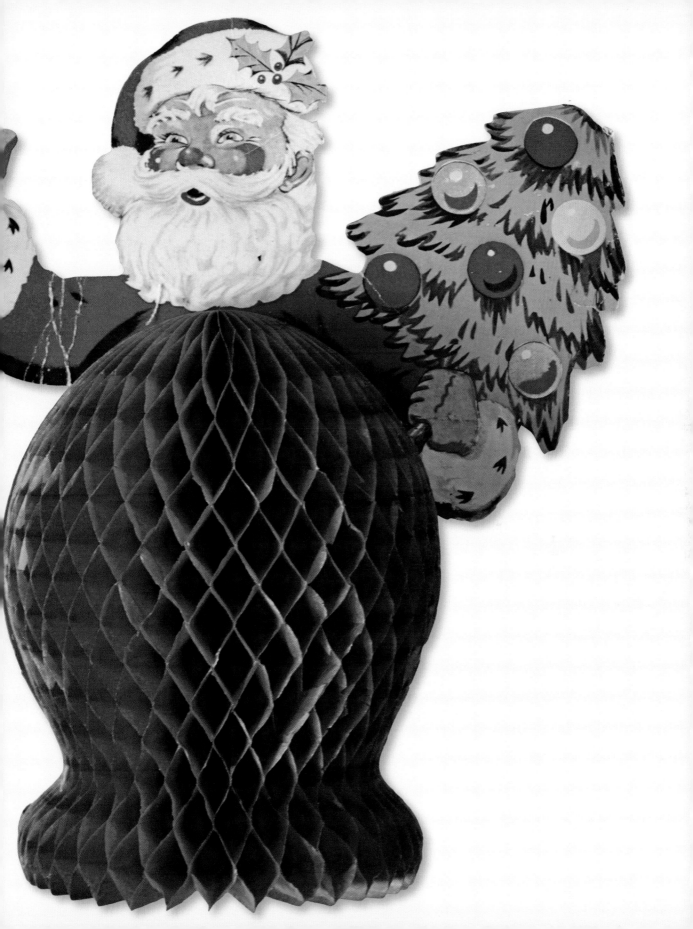

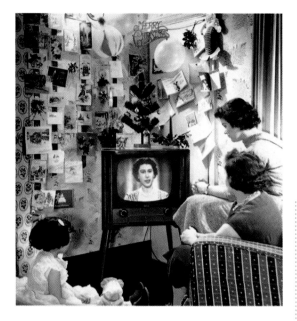

*On Christmas Day 1957,
the Queen addressed the nation
on television for the first time.*

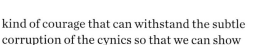

kind of courage that can withstand the subtle corruption of the cynics so that we can show the world that we are not afraid of the future.'

At one point she gestures rather expansively, as if to prove a point. She does not repeat the experiment, but keeps on going. Steadily. As she will keep on going, across the 20th century and beyond.

'It has always been easy to hate and destroy. To build and to cherish is much more difficult. That is why we can take a pride in the new Commonwealth we are building.' She ends as she always ends, wishing us all God's blessing and a Happy Christmas.

Fifty-five years later, the nation still gathers around its television sets, in a vastly different Britain – and a vastly different Commonwealth – to hear what the Queen has to say. Her rack of family photos has evolved, like every rack of family photos in the country. Her hair is white now and the film-star waist has gone, and that is what makes her annual address so apposite.

We celebrate Christmas not because it is timeless, but because it marks time. We sing old songs, we wear new clothes. We put on paper hats. Children grow up, leave home. They will love, they will have children of their own. Parents age and die. And we are reminded, every year, that all things pass and that we must cherish them while they are in our grasp.

angle, from behind an antique desk displaying family photos. Despite the blurry black-and-white camera work, there's a touch of the film star about her; she sports a tight-waisted frock of gold lamé and a helmet of dark hair. Her voice is clipped and rings like a well-behaved bell.

'Television has made it possible for many of you to see me in your homes on Christmas Day. My own family often gather round to watch television, as they are this moment, and that is how I imagine you now,' she tells her unseen audience.

The Queen acknowledges that many people find her a remote figure. 'But now, at least for a few minutes, I welcome you to the peace of my own home.' In words she has written herself, she calls for people to reclaim fundamental virtues like morality, integrity and self-restraint.

'Today we need a special kind of courage, not the kind needed in battle, but a kind which makes us stand up for everything that we know is right, everything that is true and honest. We need the

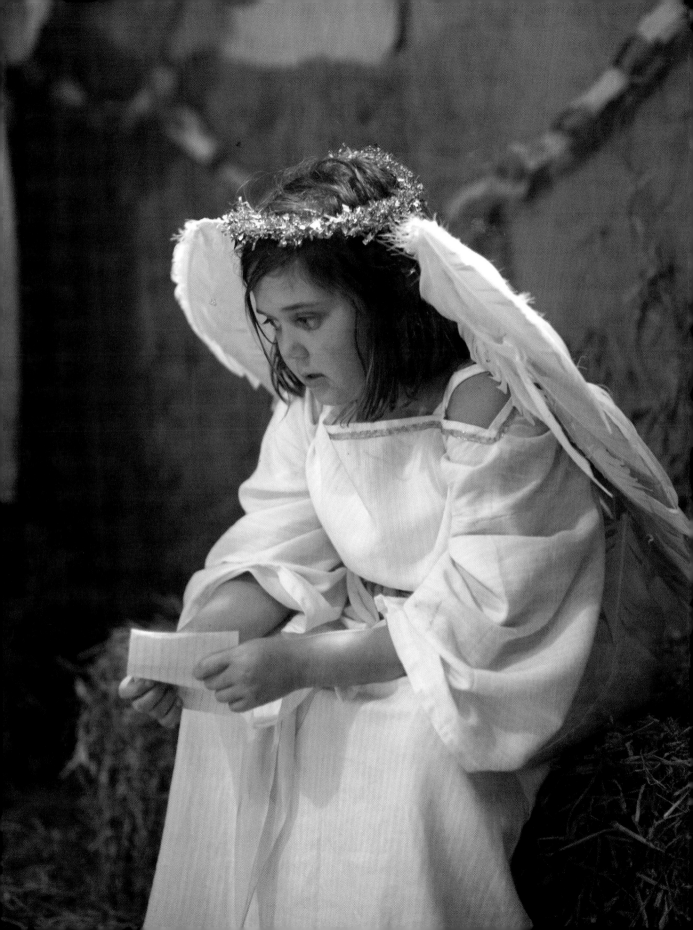

Call the Midwife

Diaries

Part 3

Jennifer takes charge, inspiring
us all - and bossing me about -
unto the end. The show surprises
everyone, and forget-me-nots bloom
in unexpected places.

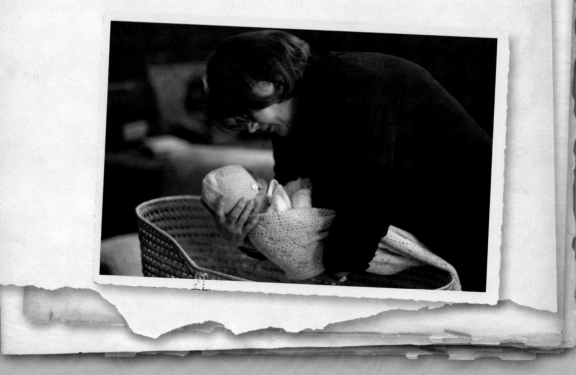

30 March 2011

I speak to Jennifer for the first time since we heard the news. Her voice is strong, which pleases me, and I find myself suddenly savouring the way she can't quite say her 'R''s. In life, small details often tell us giant truths, and it is at this moment that I realise I love her.

I don't say anything. Instead, I tell her (possibly over-brightly) all about the derelict seminary Neal Street Productions have found to film in, in Mill Hill, and that Amy is going up to Birmingham, to meet the Sisters and study a 1950s habit that they have tucked away.

When I tentatively suggest that Jennifer might like to visit us on set in June if she is feeling up to it, she simply says 'We'll see'. She doesn't elaborate, and I don't ask her to. Not for the first time in our friendship, I have to accept that she knows more than I do.

9 April 2011

Jennifer has not given notes on any of my scripts since she read the second episode, but before she was ill we often chatted on the phone. I would run things by her, and every so often she would write, with a piece of (usually random) advice.

I work on, secretly longing for a letter in her distinctive hand, perhaps petitioning for the navy coat again. But nothing comes. I speak to Philip, who says he sits by her bed and reads each new draft to her, playing all the parts.

12 April 2011

Jennifer e-mailed Pippa today, making plans for the altered way ahead. There is a shining simplicity and grace to her prose; she states that she is at peace with her diagnosis and that she considers it a case of 'Thy will be done'.

The e-mail is, above all else, a phenomenally dignified piece of literary housekeeping. Having copied in all of the relevant professionals — her agent, her publisher, Pippa, myself — Jennifer sets out, with meticulous politeness, her wishes for the series. She commends all of us to one another, and specifically states that she wants consultant midwife Terri Coates, who was her technical adviser on the books, to be her 'eyes and ears' on set.

There are a lot of clinical errors about a very premature baby, and I cannot be sure that I can accurately correct them. You need an expert, and I suggest Terri Coates, my clinical editor, whose name is at the front of the book. She has a wealth of historic knowledge, and is a practicing midwife and tutor to-day.
I can only report what I saw, & that was 55 yrs ago!!

We start filming in the middle of June. It is impossible to tell from the e-mail how long Jennifer imagines she might live. But it can't be very many months and the time she has to function normally must be dwindling by the day.

13 April 2011

Jennifer is weakening rapidly.

It is a glorious, bright blue morning, but I drive to Hemel Hempstead with a heavy heart — and a still-warm sponge cake parked on the passenger seat. I meet Pippa outside, as arranged, and all we can think of to say is, 'This is awful.'

We ring on the doorbell, and Philip shows us into his study. This had been the pattern whenever I visited, but today we don't have one of our nice chats about books or his latest painting. He looks ashen, and warns that we should stay no more than five minutes. Then he escorts us upstairs to the former guest room, where his wife is being nursed.

Jennifer's weight loss is shocking; she lies narrow as a knife in a bed no wider than a child's. A large light window, framed by a creeper, overlooks her beloved garden, which is misty with a foam of pale forget-me-nots. Philip sits by her and takes hold of her hand.

Looked after by hospice nurses and her family, Jennifer is mercifully in no pain, but querulous. Her fourth book, the book about death, has not sold well and she is of the view that this is because the publicity was poor. She wants the publicity for the series to be 'a vast improvement', and Pippa promises that this will be the case.

Talk of the show seems to give Jennifer a boost. To Philip's alarm, she gets out of bed — with the sad new accompaniment of a walking stick — to fetch a photograph album we have never seen before. It has recently been sent to her by a fellow midwife and contains page after page of snapshots from her East End days. She turns the pages with alacrity, fresh memories bubbling to the surface.

I spend a short time alone with Jennifer towards the end of the visit. Depleted by this point, and lying down again, she puts on a passable show of bossing me about, making me rearrange her get-well cards and flowers. I would be happy to do this for hours — it is her old self shining through. For as long as I aim to please, but don't quite manage it (and we both make elaborate attempts to keep our patience), everything feels much as it ever did, and not at all as though our ways are primed to part.

I fetch her some elderflower cordial, then sit by her bed and we hold hands. This is a first, as Jennifer has never been a touchy-feely sort of person. I can feel every bone in her long, slender fingers, and — without flesh to anchor them — her heavy sapphire and opal rings rotate at my gentlest touch.

We talk a little about the future of the series, and what will happen if it is a success, or not a success. In the flurry of activity surrounding pre-production, I have not yet been to visit the Sisters in Birmingham and this is something she wishes me to rectify.

'I have to say,' she says, after
a silence, 'this has all been
a rather interesting experience.'
I ask if she means the television
series or her illness. 'Both,'
she says. 'And death will be very
interesting indeed.'

It is a terrible thing to close the
door on someone you will never see
again. I leave through the dazzling
forget-me-not-filled garden (I have
never seen so many forget-me-nots)
and go out through the side gate.
I sit in my car and cry for a bit,
before acknowledging that Jennifer
would consider this impractical.
I drive home, and get on with my work.

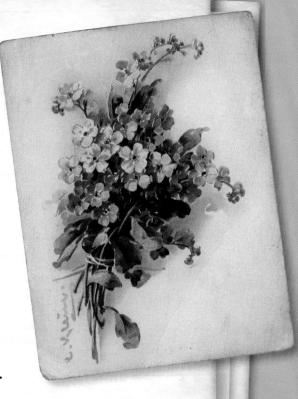

1 June 2011

I am actually working on an *Upstairs Downstairs* script when the
telephone rings. It is Philip and, as soon as I hear his voice,
my stomach lurches as there is only one reason why he would
call me now. So that he doesn't have to tell me she has gone,
I just say, 'When?' and he says, 'Yesterday.'

After I put the phone down, a hard thought hits me. I kicked
off the whole process of making *Call the Midwife* saying I would
never adapt the work of a living author. And now I'm not.

14 June 2011

To Hemel Hempstead, for Jennifer's funeral at St John's, Boxmoor. I wear a proper black mourning ensemble, which I suspect she would approve of, and high spindly heels, which I regret when I get stuck in traffic then have to park miles away, and half-run, half-stagger to the church.

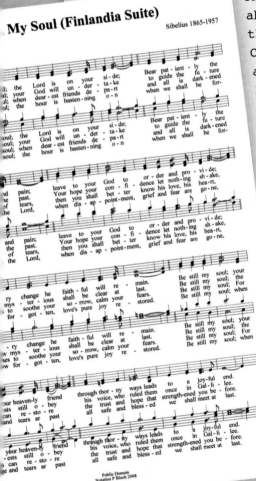

Unsurprisingly, Jennifer had clear views about the manner in which she wished to leave the world. There are no flowers and Holy Communion is part of the package. Music is also a major component. Touchingly, a choir has assembled especially for the occasion, comprising singers from ensembles with which Jennifer performed. Her grandchildren also contribute, and there are eulogies from two vicars.

The thing I find most striking is that Jennifer's late blooming as an author and her groundbreaking, bestselling books are only mentioned en passant, almost at the end of the second priest's address. I suddenly realise how small they were in the scheme of things, almost a postscript to a life that was authentic, faithful and conventional only on the surface.

The series isn't mentioned at all — until we get outside.

As Jennifer's coffin is placed in the hearse, there is some mild confusion as to whether we should follow it or go direct to the house for refreshments.

Suddenly I realise that I am in a little huddle of people whose only connection to Jennifer was through *Call the Midwife*. I am especially glad to see Tara Cook, who has been involved with all this from the start. And then Terri Coates, who has been engaged — as per Jennifer's wishes — as a consultant, bustles up, looking smart in a trouser suit. She is clutching a tear-stained tissue, but gets straight down to brass tacks.

'Heidi, I've been going over the breech birth. You're going to have to make some amendments.' And so we sit on a bench, in the sunshine and our funeral clothes, going over the delivery of the legs.

NURSING DURING LABOUR AND DELIVERY

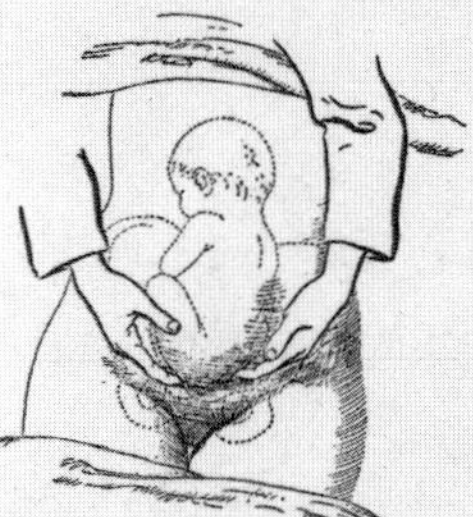

Fig. 275. First step in performing an external version.
The breech is dislodged from the pelvis.

9 September 2011

The end of the shoot is almost in sight, and I am sitting on set watching filming at Mill Hill. It's a scene in the bike shed with Jenny and Jimmy. She is supposed to be telling him she doesn't love him, but one of the bicycles keeps unintentionally falling over, and we've all got the giggles, which doesn't assist the mood.

Between takes, while someone tries to mend the bicycle, I wander off to pick a few blackberries. The brambles grow all around the seminary grounds and over the graves of the Jesuits who are buried there. It occurs to me that for a show that's supposed to be about new life, *Call the Midwife* seems rather content to walk hand in hand with those no longer with us.

There's a frail wild rose, almost spent, growing over a bit of broken fence. I am suddenly reminded that there is actually a rose created in honour of the Royal College of Midwives, called 'Breath of Life'. It's an apricot-coloured climber, and I think how nice it would be if Pippa and I planted one here before we leave, in memory of Jennifer who brought us to this place.

And then I stumble across a vast swathe of such irresistible blackberries that I have to go off and find a bowl to put them in.

28 September 2011

Today is the final day of filming. I won't be able to go to the party tonight, because I have to drive to Cardiff for the *Upstairs Downstairs* readthrough. I did, however, get my end-of-term present in the post this morning. It is a novelty condom, which I have little use for and place proudly on the mantelpiece.

I am packing the car, when my phone pings with a text. It is from Hugh, our producer 'Just wrapped. All done. Very emotional.' And I kick myself, because we never got round to planting that rose for Jennifer at Mill Hill, and now we've missed our chance and it will not come again.

16 January 2012

The first episode of *Call the Midwife* went out last night. At 8pm.

We were all deeply worried when we heard about the time slot. Pippa and I wrote a number of e-mails expressing our concerns, but the plan did not change. I'm convinced that people will have turned off in their droves. We have shots of babies' heads emerging, syphilis, a haemorrhage and a rather cheerful enema. It is hardly pre-watershed fare — and we've already been told that men won't watch it, young women won't watch it, and pregnant women won't watch it. Who on earth *will* watch it?

I have decided I don't want to know the viewing figures. They usually come in at about 10am, and I busy myself with other things, like making a Bakewell tart. Only when the landline has been ringing and the mobile pinging for an hour do I decide I'd better check my messages.

Over eight million. Bigger even than *Cranford*, bigger than anything for years. But not big enough because all the viewers in the world can't bridge the gulf between this moment and the friend I want to phone.

Overnight viewing figures: OVER 8 MILLION!!

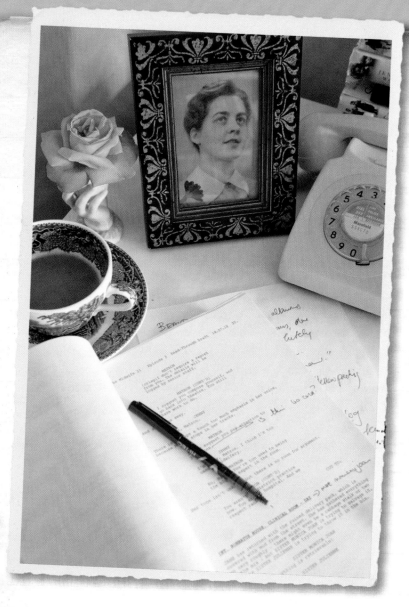

I look at Jennifer's picture, the one I keep by my computer, where I can see it when I'm writing. And for some daft and random reason, I am reminded of the gypsy woman and her bunch of suspect heather. Telling me my life would change on the fifteenth of the month.

Postscript

The figures for the *Call the Midwife* series went up and up, week by week, peaking at over 11.4 million. Pippa e-mailed the morning after the second episode was broadcast: the BBC had already asked for another series. The show became a sort of national phenomenon, and Jennifer's books — which had always sold steadily — went whizzing back up to the top of the charts. Even *In the Midst of Life*, the book about death whose poor sales had so grieved her, made it into the Top Ten. I suspected she would find this gratifying.

But I still had a nagging feeling that one last sign or gesture was required. As we were making plans to return to Mill Hill, I thought perhaps I would buy that 'Breath of Life' rose, and plant it in the grounds when we went back.

I was spared the trouble when — a year to the day after our final conversation — I took a break from writing and went outside into my own small garden. There, self-seeded by some accident of nature, was a clump of foaming pale forget-me-nots.

I filled a vase with them and placed it on my desk by Jennifer's photograph. I hesitate to say this closed the circle, but in some mute, inexpressible way, it made things feel complete. One way or another, the link between us will remain. We are in this together, just as we always were.

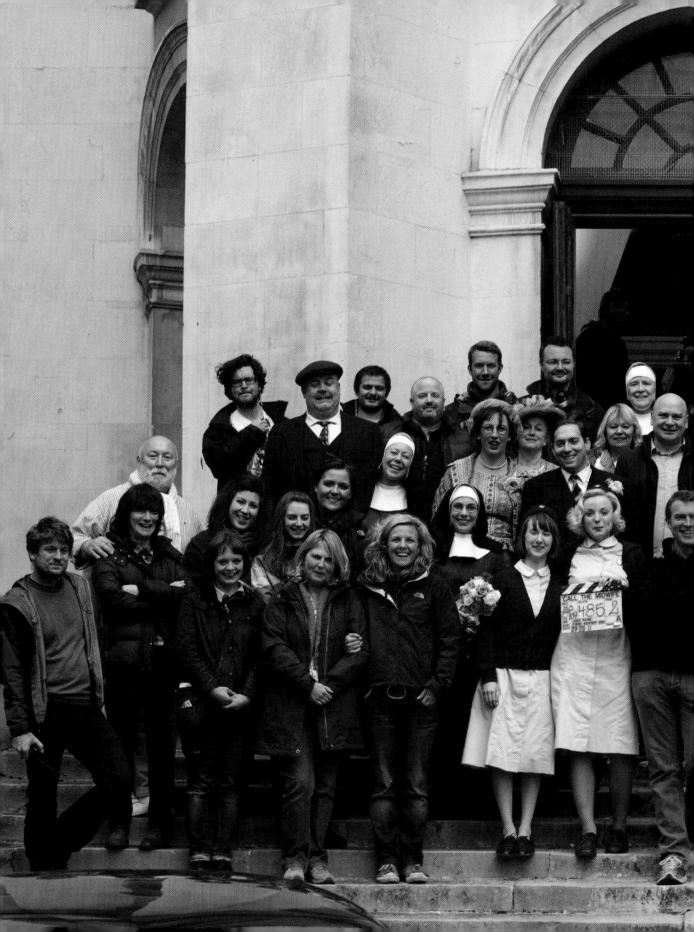

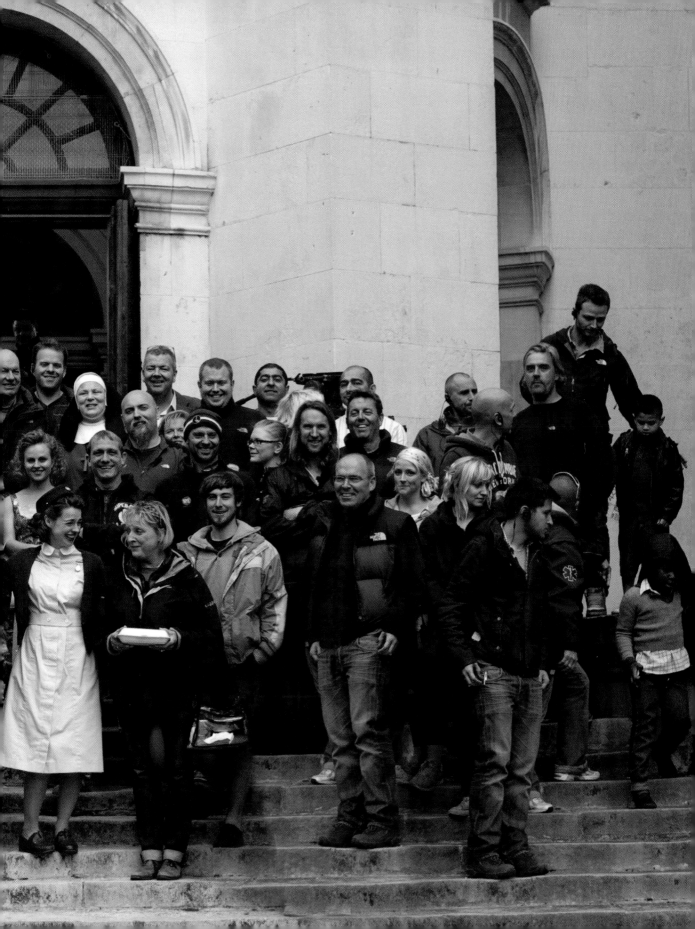

CAST AND CREW – SERIES 1

MAIN CAST

Jenny Lee	*Jessica Raine*
Sister Julienne	*Jenny Agutter*
Sister Evangelina	*Pam Ferris*
Chummy Browne	*Miranda Hart*
Sister Monica Joan	*Judy Parfitt*
Trixie Franklin	*Helen George*
Cynthia Miller	*Bryony Hannah*
Sister Bernadette	*Laura Main*
Fred	*Cliff Parisi*
Dr Turner	*Stephen McGann*
PC Peter Noakes	*Ben Caplan*
Jimmy	*George Rainsford*
Mature Jennifer (voice over)	*Vanessa Redgrave*

MAIN CREW

Series created and written by	*Heidi Thomas*
Writers	*Harriet Warner*
	Jack Williams
	Esther Wilson
Directors	*Philippa Lowthorpe*
	Jamie Payne
Producer	*Hugh Warren*
Casting Director	*Andy Pryor CDG*
Consultant Midwife	*Terri Coates RM*
Location Manager	*Antonia Grant*
First Assistant Directors	*Toni Staples*
	Nick Brown
Post Production Supervisor	*Heidi Mount*
Co-Producer	*Tara Cook*
Sound Recordist	*Rudi Buckle*
Make-Up & Hair Designer	*Christine Walmesley-Cotham*
Costume Designer	*Amy Roberts*
Editors	*David Thrasher*
	Jamie Trevill
Composer	*Peter Salem*
Director of Photography	*Chris Seager BSC*
Production Designer	*Eve Stewart*
Line Producer	*Patrick Schweitzer*
Executive Producers	*Pippa Harris*
	Heidi Thomas

GUEST ARTISTS – SERIES 1

EPISODE ONE

Len Warren	*Tim Faraday*
Conchita Warren	*Carolina Validés*
Maureen Warren	*Hayley Squires*
Pearl Winston	*Lorraine Stanley*
Mrs Hawkes	*Lacey Bond*
Muriel	*Sarah Ridgeway*
Eddy	*Benjamin Wilkin*
Registrar	*David Annen*

EPISODE TWO

Father Joe	*Stanley Townsend*
Ingrid Mason	*Sophie Cosson*
Clifford Mason	*Liam Reilly*
Mary	*Amy McAllister*
Zakir	*Darwin Shaw*
Charmaine	*Jessica Jones*
Sailor	*Mitchell Hunt*
Jack Smith	*Jake Bailey*
Betty Smith	*Victoria Alcock*
Mr Smith	*Nick Bartlett*
Mrs Fraser	*Amelda Brown*
Brenda McEntee	*Penny Layden*
Café Proprietor	*Terry Bird*

EPISODE THREE

Joe Collett	*Roy Hudd*
Winnie Lawson	*Tessa Churchard*
Ted Lawson	*John Ashton*
Officer	*David Maybrick*
Neighbour	*Valerie King*

EPISODE FOUR

Shirley Redmond	*Emma Noakes*
Ron Redmond	*Tom Colley*
Gladys	*Susie Baxter*
David Jones	*Tom Goodman-Hill*
Margaret Jones	*Thomasin Rand*
Eileen	*Nicola Munns*
Milkman	*Anton Saunders*

EPISODE FIVE

Frank	*Sean Baker*
Peggy	*Elizabeth Rider*
Tip	*Jake Davies*
Elsie May	*Sarah Counsell*
Barry May	*Brett Allen*
Mrs Leonard	*Candis Nergaard*

EPISODE SIX

Cakey Crumb	*Jeff Innocent*
Cathy Powell	*Tina O'Brien*
Lady Fortescue-Browne	*Cheryl Campbell*
Chairman	*Robin Browne*
Mrs Leck	*Debra Baker*
Jesu Emanuel	*Kika Markham*
Sergeant Parry	*John Vernon*
Mr Briggs	*Graham Padden*
Mrs Foster	*Elizabeth Webster*

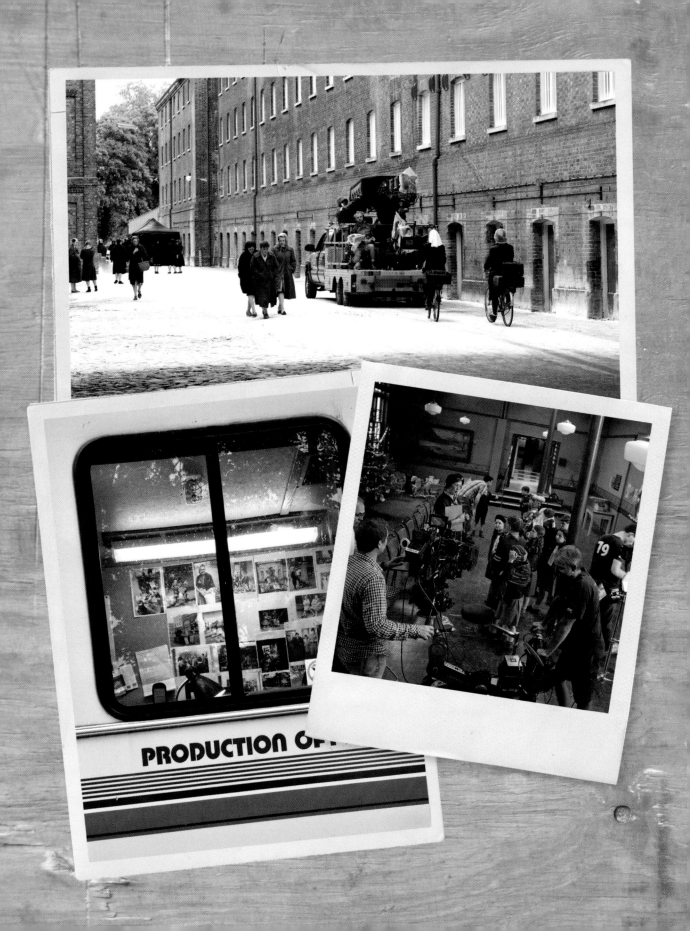

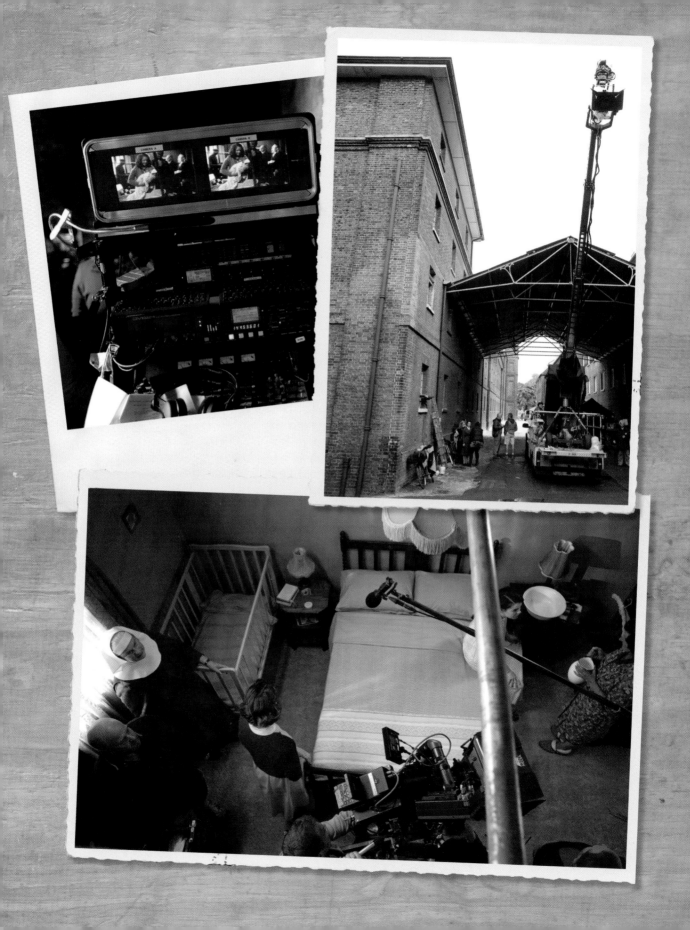

THE ARCHITECTS

JENNIFER WORTH AUTHOR

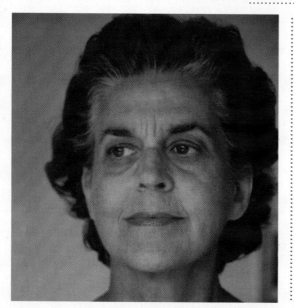

Best-selling author Jennifer Worth was born in Clacton-on-Sea in 1935 and grew up in the Buckinghamshire town of Amersham. She trained as a nurse at the Royal Berkshire Hospital in Reading, then moved to London to study midwifery. In the 1950s she worked as a midwife in Poplar, east London, where she lived with the Anglican Community of St John the Divine, who play a central part in her trilogy of *Call the Midwife* memoirs under the psuedonym of the 'midwives of St Raymund Nonnatus'. After 20 years of nursing, she left the profession to embark on a musical career, becoming a licenciate of the London College of Music in 1974. She was awarded a fellowship ten years later, and taught piano and singing for over 25 years. Jennifer died in May 2011, leaving her husband Philip, two daughters and three grandchildren.

PIPPA HARRIS EXECUTIVE PRODUCER

Pippa Harris, Executive Producer on *Call the Midwife*, established Neal Street Productions in 2003, with Sam Mendes and Caro Newling, and runs the Film and TV division. Prior to this she was the BBC's Head of Drama Commissioning. Since forming the company, Pippa has produced *Starter For Ten*, co-produced *Jarhead* and co-executive produced Sam Mendes' *Revolutionary Road*. Recent successes include the critically acclaimed BBC Two Shakespeare mini-series, *The Hollow Crown*, which she executive produced. On bringing Jennifer Worth's books to life, Pippa says, 'The books were brought to my attention by my Neal Street colleague, Tara Cook, when *Call the Midwife* was published in 2007. We were scouting for film projects, but *Call the Midwife* cried out to be a TV series. It was the mixture of wonderful characters, gripping storylines and the combination of humour and pathos that made me think it would work well on TV.'

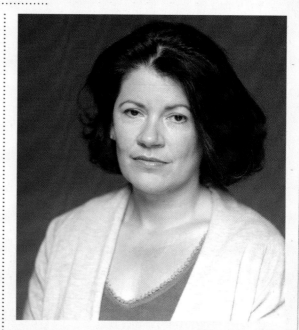

HUGH WARREN *PRODUCER*

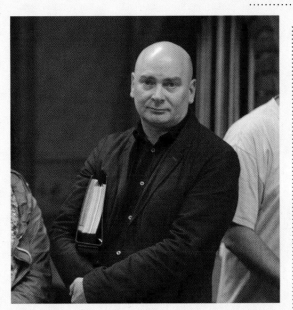

Hugh began his career as a producer in 1999 with the BAFTA nominated BBC series *Playing the Field*. Since then, Hugh has gone on to produce a range of drama series including *Above Suspicion: Deadly Intent*, *Survivors*, *Bonkers*, *The Chase*, *Blue Murder* and *At Home with the Braithwaites*. Hugh has also produced several television movies such as the BAFTA-nominated *Doctor Zhivago* with Keira Knightley, *The Best Man*, *Suspicion* and *Frankenstein*. Hugh is proud of the emotional honesty of *Call the Midwife*: 'I believe we have been faithful to the spirit of Jennifer's books. Childbirth is inherently dramatic and full of heightened emotions, but the stories Jennifer recounts in the books also contain universal themes of love and redemption which provide a resonance and truth that are timeless. They're unflinching yet life-enhancing stories.'

PHILIPPA LOWTHORPE *DIRECTOR*

Philippa Lowthorpe, Principal Director of *Call the Midwife*, is an award-winning film maker, who began her career making documentaries for the BBC. Her credits include cult documentary *Three Salons at the Seaside*, *A Childhood* and *Remember the Family*. Her drama credits include the highly acclaimed BBC film *The Other Boleyn Girl*, *Sex, The City and Me* and *Five Daughters*, which won several awards including Prix Europa and the RTS Society award for Best Drama. Of the *Call the Midwife* series, she says, 'I love stories about real people, and I love stories about women which are unearthed from an unknown history. This project had both elements. These midwives and nuns are truly unsung heroines. The work they did in the East End was amazing and no one has ever celebrated that before... I also adore Heidi Thomas's writing. She's captured the world so brilliantly.'

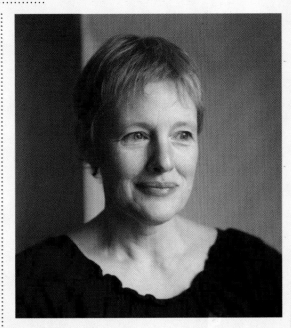

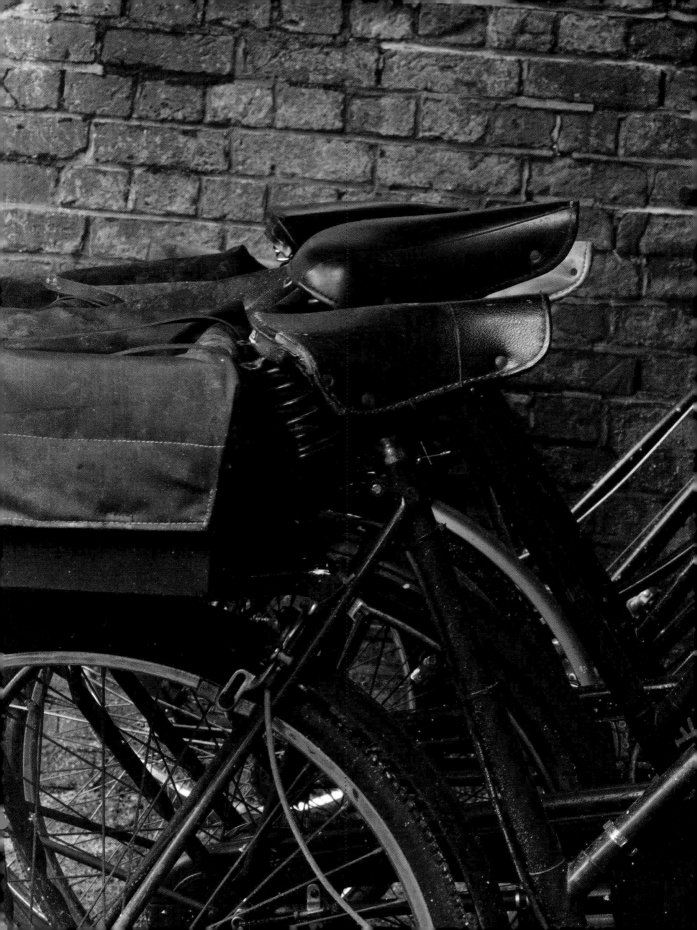

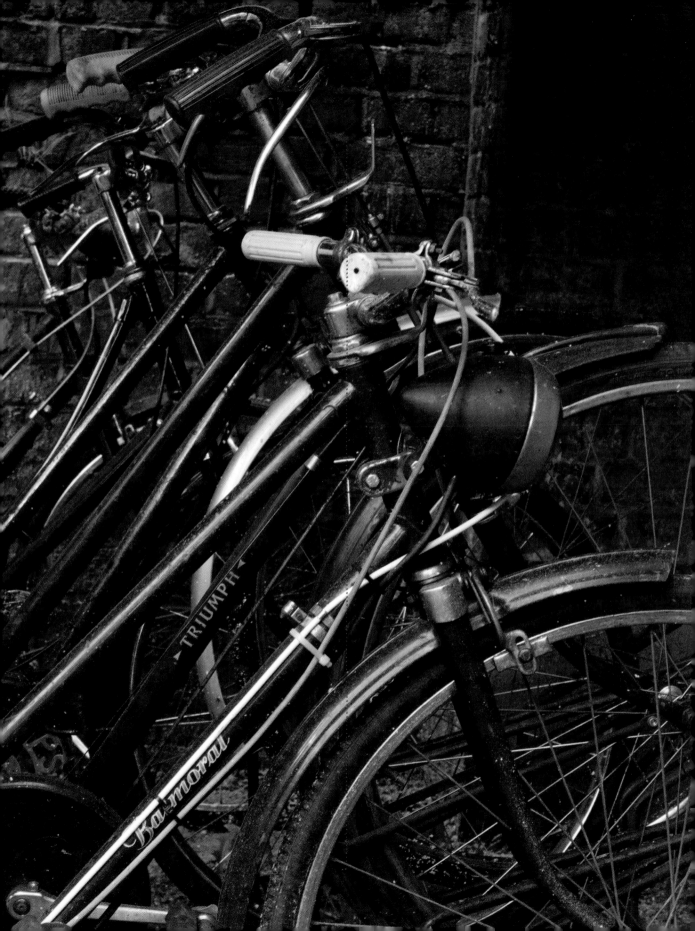

PICTURE CREDITS

178–179 background; 179 bottom right; 180 background, top right; 186–187; 191; 192 bottom; 197 background; 198–199 background; 216–217 (background); 223 hats; 229 top left, bottom right; 232–233; 248–249 background; 261

COURTESY OF WOOLWORTHSMUSEUM.CO.UK
Pg 93 background

REPRODUCED WITH GRATEFUL THANKS TO
THE FAMILY OF JENNIFER WORTH
Pg 100; 104; 106; 165; 266; 282 top

Pg 90 top (jellyfann.com)
Pg 121 bottom (BPM Media)
Pg 113 top right (The Community of St John the Divine
Pg 150 top left; 153 middle image (Courtesy of NHS
Scotland)
Pg 184 left (Sarah Bealby-Wright)
Pg 253 top left (Rupert Bear®: © 2012 Classic Media
Distribution Limited and Express Newspapers. All Rights
Reserved / Courtesy of Rupert the Bear Annuals)
Pg 283 bottom (Huntley Hedworth)

While every effort has been made to trace the owners
of copyright material reproduced herein and secure
permissions, the publishers would like to apologise for
any omissions and will be pleased to incorporate missing
acknowledgements in any future edition of this book.

AUTHOR'S ACKNOWLEDGEMENTS
From conception through to delivery, the *Call
The Midwife Companion* has been a labour of love
for many very special people, and Pippa Harris and
I are indebted to them all.

Our sincere thanks go to Annabel Merullo, Bethan
Evans, and Hannah MacDonald, who did so much to
get the project up and running. We are also extremely
grateful to the entire cast and crew of the *Call the Midwife* series – especially Jenny Agutter, Terri Coates, Amy
Roberts, Eve Stewart, Christine Walmesley-Cotham and
Hugh Warren – for being so generous with their precious
time and energy.

Graphic design team We Are Laura have our love and
admiration for their exquisite art work, as does Laurence
Cendrowicz for his gorgeous photographs.

Affectionate gratitude also goes to *Call The Midwife*'s
original BBC Executive Producer Sarah Brandist, whose
own maternal journey prevented her from seeing the
show through to its birth; to Philip Worth and Suzannah
Hart, for their grace and continued friendship, and to
the Community of St John the Divine for their kindness,
hospitality and prayers.

We would also like to thank the book's magnificent
midwives – our glorious researcher Karen Farrington
and wonderful editor Laura Nickoll – along with its
redoubtable godfather, Iain MacGregor.

PUBLISHER'S ACKNOWLEDGEMENTS
Collins would like to thank the following for their
help: Tower Hamlets Archives, The Royal College of
Midwives, Emma Callery, Ian Johnson Publicity and
Caroline Reynolds.

Publishing Director: Iain MacGregor
Art Director: Martin Topping
Designers: We Are Laura
Project Editor: Laura Nickoll
Editorial Assistant: Chloe Slattery

The Life and Times of Call the Midwife
The Official Companion to Seasons One and Two

First published in the United Kingdom in 2012 by Collins, an imprint of HarperCollins*Publishers*

HarperCollins books may be purchased for educational, business, or sales promotional use. For information please write: Special Markets Department, HarperCollins*Publishers*, 10 East 53rd Street, New York, NY 10022.

Harper Design
An Imprint of HarperCollins*Publishers*
10 East 53rd Street
New York, NY 10022
Tel: (212) 207-7000
Fax: (212) 207-7654

Text written by Heidi Thomas
Principal set photographer: Laurence Cendrowicz

Call the Midwife
A Neal Street Production for the BBC

ISBN 978-0-06-225003-2

Printed in the United States of America
First printing, 2012

1 3 5 7 9 10 8 6 4 2

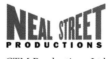

CTM Productions Ltd

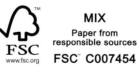

MIX
Paper from
responsible sources
FSC C007454

FSC™ is a non-profit international organisation established to promote the responsible management of the world's forests. Products carrying the FSC label are independently certified to assure consumers that they come from forests that are managed to meet the social, economic and ecological needs of present and future generations, and other controlled sources.

Find out more about HarperCollins and the environment at
www.harpercollins.com